"COVID-19 exposed how our unequal societ[   ] health. In his new book, Stephen Bezruchk[   ] of the problem, and makes a case for the changes necessary for creating a healthier world."

Sandro Galea,
Dean School of Public Health, Boston University

"Capitalism, as Piketty showed us again, generates and deepens inequality. Bezruchka's book shows us how that inequality shortens lives across the world even among those who celebrate capitalism. This important book also drives home a crucial lesson for public health we need to draw from our very diverse COVID experiences."

Richard D. Wolff,
Professor of Economics Emeritus, University of Massachusetts,
Amherst, and co-founder of Democracy at Work

"When the pandemic hit, we imagined a silver lining—'at least we'll realize that we're in this together.' That laughable naiveté evaporated as the virus disproportionately savaged America's have-nots. Stephen Bezruchka, one of the subject's wisest scholars, documents how COVID-19 is merely a sped-up version of decades of festering health inequality. This superb book will convince anyone other than ideologues that something is brutally wrong with American health."

Robert Sapolsky,
Professor of Biology, and Professor of Neurology
and of Neurosurgery, Stanford University

"*Inequality Kills Us All* diagnoses nations as if they were patients, showing how poverty and riches are both human inventions that come with serious public health consequences. The always insightful and provocative Stephen Bezruchka was an emergency physician who then taught Nepali doctors in remote areas there before becoming a public health professor. He teaches how policy choices determine longevity and quality of life, and how smarter policies would reduce harm while spreading more joy."

David Cay Johnston,
Pulitzer Prize-winning investigative reporter
and bestselling author

"This book should be a must-read for politicians, policymakers, and the public. It shows how and why the COVID-19 pandemic wrought such havoc in America, and how inequality set the scene for that chaos and is the biggest public health challenge of our time. We ignore the evidence assembled so skillfully here at our peril."

Kate E. Pickett,

Professor of Epidemiology, Deputy Director of the Centre for Future Health, Associate Director of the Leverhulme Centre for Anthropocene Biodiversity, University of York

"In the midst of a public health crisis of unimaginable magnitude, Stephen Bezruchka diagnoses the central, interlocked issues—from biological to social—that explain how and why the COVID-19 pandemic manifested in the United States, with many lessons for countries around the world. His autopsy of the pandemic provides a clear sense that those in power should feel shame about the role that politics has played both in developing the longstanding conditions that primed society to experience a highly unequal pandemic and in delivering at best an anemic response during the pandemic. It also gives a clear-eyed sense of the way forward, should we heed the messages provided throughout this important book."

Arjumand Siddiqi,

Professor and Canada Research Chair in Population Health Equity, Dalla Lana School of Public Health, University of Toronto

"The moribund patient is the American population. The disease is structural violence. Bezruchka has been tracking US vital signs for over three decades. Our symptoms are centuries old with unaddressed institutional inequities, cultures of rigged meritocracy, over-consumption, greed, and waste for the few, but under-service, overwork, under-pay, disenfranchisement, and invisibility for the many. The tragic, ongoing dual pandemic of COVID failure and systemic racial violence has brought all this to light. *Inequality Kills Us All* presents diagnostic and preventative medicine we cannot do without. Bezruchka reminds us that our social ills, health crises, and political breakdowns are ineffably intertwined. Our solutions must also be collective, cooperative, and from the ground up. Let this brilliant volume of evidence-based medicine for the body politic begin our collective resuscitation."

Rachel R. Chapman,

Associate Professor, Department of Anthropology, University of Washington

Inequality Kills Us All

The complex answer to why the United States does so poorly in health meas-ures has at its base one pervasive issue: The United States has by far the highest levels of inequality of all the rich countries. *Inequality Kills Us All* details how living in a society with entrenched hierarchies increases the negative effects of illnesses for everyone.

The antidote must start, Stephen Bezruchka recognizes, with a broader awareness of the nature of the problem, and out of that understanding policies that eliminate these inequalities: A fair system of taxation, so that the rich are paying their share; support for child well-being, including paid parental leave, continued monthly child support payments, and equitable educational opportunities; universal access to healthcare; and a guaranteed income for all Americans. The aim is to have a society that treats everyone well—and health will follow.

Stephen Bezruchka is Associate Teaching Professor Emeritus in the Depart-ments of Health Systems & Population Health and of Global Health at the School of Public Health, University of Washington, in Seattle. He worked as an emergency physician for decades and now teaches the concepts presented in this book at the University of Washington.

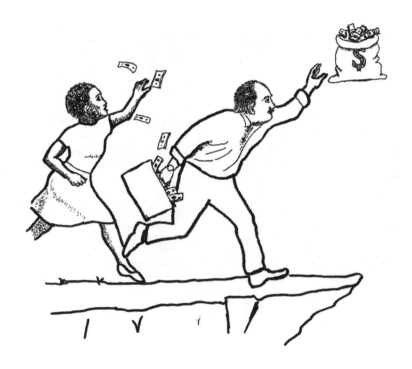

Inequality Kills Us All

COVID-19's Health Lessons for the World

Stephen Bezruchka

To Mary
For our health!
Stephen

Routledge
Taylor & Francis Group

NEW YORK AND LONDON

Cover image: Shutterstock, ArtMari
Opposite Title Page art by Lon Rosen

First published 2023
by Routledge
605 Third Avenue, New York, NY 10158

and by Routledge
2 Park Square, Milton Park, Abingdon, Oxon, OX14 4RN

Routledge is an imprint of the Taylor & Francis Group, an informa business

© 2023 Taylor & Francis

Library of Congress Cataloging-in-Publication Data
Names: Bezruchka, Stephen, author.
Title: Inequality kills us all : COVID-19's health lessons for the world /
    Stephen Bezruchka.
Description: New York, NY : Routledge, 2022. | Includes bibliographical
    references and index.
Identifiers: LCCN 2022021080 | ISBN 9781032326214 (hardback) | ISBN
    9781032278391 (paperback) | ISBN 9781003315889 (ebook)
Subjects: LCSH: Public health--United States. | Health services
    accessibility--United States. | Medical care--Political aspects--United
    States. | Equality--Health apsects--United States | COVID-19 Pandemic,
    2020---Social aspects--United States.
Classification: LCC RA445 .B49 2022 | DDC
    362.1962/41400973--dc23/eng/20220803
LC record available at https://lccn.loc.gov/2022021080

ISBN: 978-1-032-32621-4 (hbk)
ISBN: 978-1-032-27839-1 (pbk)
ISBN: 978-1-003-31588-9 (ebk)

DOI: 10.4324/9781003315889

Typeset in Garamond
by KnowledgeWorks Global Ltd.

To all those who died of social murder or structural violence.

Contents

Acknowledgments

Some books have a short gestation. A concept, a few months' work, and it is done. So, it was in 1988 with a manual I wrote on travel medicine. *Inequality Kills Us All* has taken more than a quarter of a century to be born. In 1991, fertilization occurred on a rice paddy in remote eastern Nepal, where my course on population health for medical students and doctors took place. My Nepali co-leader, Dr. Shankar Man Rai, asked me why Bangladeshi men had better survival than men in Harlem, New York. He had read a 1990 paper in the *New England Journal of Medicine* presenting that data. I was clueless.

Another development was in 1995, after completing my public health degree. I began my transition from doctoring individuals to wanting to make a population healthy. I presented ideas from this book to conferences of doctors then, somehow thinking those in my profession were interested in health as well as medical care. My first draft of a book proposal followed the next year. After encouraging rejections from agents, I focused on writing shorter pieces for newspapers and magazines. By the turn of the millennium, I found my niche teaching courses on population health in the School of Public Health at the University of Washington.

My greatest critic, supporter, and editor became my wife, Mary Anne Mercer, whom I met while pursuing the MPH degree at Johns Hopkins University. My most profound teachers have been my children, Michael Bezruchka and Maia Mercer.

I had to be an autodidact in the emerging field of population health. I gained confidence to present valid material in whatever venue by getting to know the leaders in this nascent field. Spending considerable time with Richard Wilkinson, Ichiro Kawachi, and Clyde Hertzman sharpened my critical thinking skills. I had the fortune to spend a month with Richard in Nepal in 1999. I had already spent quite a few years there and thought I could respond to most questions. Richard Wilkinson's observations and critical thinking skills challenged me to see much there I wasn't aware of.

For those who were deceased, such as John Bowlby, I found people who had spent considerable time with them. Dennis Raphael shared his experiences and energy. Attending scientific conferences where the book's ideas were presented and discussed gave me valuable insight. The early life concepts were not main-stream, but meeting with David Barker and attending international meet-ings on the developmental origins of health and disease gave me confidence that these ideas had scientific validity. A contemporary, Gregg Bennett, who attended my graduate course as a non-student (a term I learned in Berkeley in the early 1970s), was motivated by my thinking on medical harm and wanted to collaborate on a book. We had a manuscript draft by 2010, but no publisher. Teaching, other writing, and talking presented convenient distractions.

The best way to understand something is to teach it. Richard Wilkinson and Kate Pickett wrote *The Spirit Level*, which became the textbook for my courses. They remain lifelong friends. I learned much from the thinking of my relatively unconstrained students, who voiced the phrase "early life lasts a lifetime." When I talked about cells, individuals, and populations, a student remarked, insightfully, that medical care "treats cells" rather than whole persons. Coining phrases such as the Health Olympics solidified ideas. Teaching this material to groups ranging from elementary school students to those in retirement homes required vastly different strategies. While you could present slide images on screen to college students, more active learning methods were required for younger folk. Personal stories are the best for retirees.

My parents, Jaroslaw and Stefania, let me follow my own path and were always there when I needed them. As I reflect on those who have profoundly influenced my thinking on matters of health and politics and led me to various paths, profound thanks must go to: John Antrobus, David Barsamian, Noam Chomsky, Roy Little, Elizabeth Matthews, Ralph Nader, Carl Offner, David Payne, Lon Rosen, and Fred Zimmerman.

Many others helped gestate this book including Rachel Chapman, Ben Danielson, Andra DeVoght, Hailey Dowling, Steve Gloyd, Linn Gould, Amy Hagopian, Julian Perez, James Pfeiffer, and Sam Pizzigati. The myriad stu-dents I have had the privilege to teach concepts in this book deserve the great-est acknowledgment. My colleagues at the University of Washington have been very supportive. Thank you all.

Effective teaching at any level requires crafting exercises appropriate for the subject material. For high school students, a readers' theater staging of the Health Olympics entertained and engaged students. College students had to present what they learned to a group of others, which became community outreach exercises. Initially, I had them screen a segment of the Public Broadcasting Service documentary series, "Unnatural Causes: Is Inequality Making Us Sick?" followed up with a discussion. When physical distancing became the norm with COVID-19 and indoor venues were shuttered, social media provided a much broader audience than was ever possible in a single room.

In 2017, I began again in earnest, searching for people who espoused the ideas in this book. Sandro Galea, the Dean of the School of Public Health at Boston University, became a great role model. Most people who will present the poor health status of Americans were typically not born in the United States but gained insight after coming here.

Chuck Collins, a friend for many years, referred me to Dean Birkenkamp, an editor at Routledge, who was very enthusiastic about my proposal. Tom Miller became my agent to guide me through the publishing maze. Janice Harper was always available to skillfully edit the contents. Adam Hoverman and Howard Waitzkin offered critical review.

There are very many books published annually that sell few copies. P.T. Barnum, the circus giant, said: "without promotion, something terrible happens.....NOTHING." Thanks to Lorna Garano for her marketing and publicity work.

The killing fields of inequality can be overcome but only if we fight them together.

Foreword

Scientific research on questions such as whether or not income inequality causes ill health and higher death rates is no less scientific because it has important and sensitive political implications. But findings in similar areas, such as on the causes of health inequalities, are often treated as if their political importance makes them less scientific. The major political, religious, and personal battles around some of the most important scientific theories—think of Darwin, Copernicus, or Galileo—are well known. So too among the scientists proposing different interpretations of relativity or quantum mechanics in the first half of the twentieth century, who often had a huge sense of personal investment and commitment to their theories. That scientists may be deeply invested in their different theories makes their theories no less scientific. As philosophers of science, such as Professor Sir Karl Popper, have pointed out, it is not the sources of scientific theories—the scientists themselves—who need to be unbiased, it is the methods of testing those theories.

During my career, I have had the privilege of seeing research on the relationship between income inequality and health progress from its controversial beginnings to being established as fact. The link has now been tested literally hundreds of times around the world in different contexts by researchers using different controls and publishing their findings in peer-reviewed journals. Now that the dust from early controversies has settled and the scientific conclusions are clear, we need politicians, policymakers, and the public to understand it. Without that follow-up, the research is stillborn.

Stephen Bezruchka was one of the first people to recognize the importance of this research and to incorporate it in his writing and broadcasting, as well as in his teaching of medical and public health students and the wider public. What makes him a good communicator—and he has won several awards for the quality of his teaching and communication—is that his remarkable range of experience and education has given him a deep understanding of the issues and an originality of thought.

Both Stephen's parents were migrants from Ukraine to Canada. His father was a cobbler, and his mother cleaned hotel rooms until marriage and childcare.

Stephen was brought up above the family's shoe repair shop in Toronto. From a first degree in Mathematics and Physics in Toronto, he went on to a higher degree in Math at Harvard. He qualified in medicine at Stanford and in public health at Johns Hopkins University. He spent years in Nepal and was part of the first Canadian Everest expedition, but was particularly interested in its people and culture. He learned Nepali, worked on and directed healthcare projects in rural areas, and wrote what is still often regarded as the best book on trekking in Nepal.

For close to 25 years, Stephen worked in emergency medicine in Seattle, which he combined with university teaching at the University of Washington. Working in the emergency room of a big city hospital reveals, on a daily basis, the underside, the seamy side, of society—the victims of violence, self-harm, drug overdoses, alcohol addiction, accidents, and mental illness. It is where the heavy burden and high costs of our social system are most evident. This book and its many insights reflect that extraordinarily rich and varied background.

The author takes the United States as his patient and shows us why the USA has lower life expectancy than almost all other rich developed societies; why, despite spending so much more on medical care than other countries, it nevertheless fails to match their health; why the USA has suffered a much higher death rate from COVID-19 than most other rich countries; and why its life expectancy has, since before the pandemic, been declining—again, in contrast to most rich countries. Although he points out the many failings of the USA, Bezruchka's motive is an expression of his caring for the country and his desire for it to do as well as he knows it could. But you cannot heal patients without first exploring the extent and nature of their injuries. Although that is where Bezruchka starts, this is not a mere academic text: He seeks the reader's practical involvement in coaxing the patient back to health. Unlike other books on public health, he not only suggests policy prescriptions, but ends with an extraordinarily good discussion of what each of us can do to make our voices heard and turn things around.

Medicine and public health are a particularly good place from which to try to understand a society. Health is not only affected by material circumstances, such as housing, diet, and air pollution, but also by psychosocial factors including social status, social relationships, and feelings of self-worth and of whether or not we feel valued. These circumstances affect health primarily through chronic stress, making us more vulnerable to a wide range of diseases—so much so that its long-term effects look much like more rapid ageing. And rather than depending simply on subjective measures of some of these factors, they can be tracked by a number of objective biological markers of stress.

So in place of the overly materialistic view of much of economics, which often seems blind to the problems of social life and of the prevailing social structures, an understanding of the determinants of health gives us an insight into both the material and psychological problems of a society and how it impacts the population. Given that the patient is the United States and its shorter life expectancy and higher COVID-19 deaths rates—compared to almost all other rich countries—are not its only problems, this is crucially important. The USA also has much higher homicide rates and incarceration rates, more drug deaths and obesity, and children with lower levels of well-being and lower average math and literacy scores than most other rich countries. My own country, the UK, runs it a close second on several of these outcomes. Together, these factors are merely other symptoms of the patient's condition, and it is true to say that if the quality of life was higher, its length would be longer.

It is hard not to be fearful for the future of the United States, given how polarized its politics have become. But there is now good evidence that the extent of economic inequality is one of the most important drivers of that polarization, and it is that inequality which lies at the center of Bezruchka's analysis. Turning a society around is like turning a very large ship: It takes time. These problems cannot be solved in just a couple of years, even with the best political will and policy. And as well as addressing the health issues which are the focus of this book, we know that making the transition to environmental sustainability is essential to future of humanity.

Societies work best and are most adaptable when they are united, but the evidence makes it very clear that economic inequality increases the importance of class and status, and of superiority and inferiority, reducing trust and social cohesion. If we are to get through a difficult period, Bezruchka's analysis needs to be widely read and acted upon.

Professor Richard Wilkinson,
Social Epidemiologist, Co founder of the Equality Trust

Introduction

The U.S. Federal Government reports that our lives have been more disrupted with COVID-19 than any preceding event since World War II. Our interactions with others, the work we do, and the ways we get around and communicate, almost every aspect of our lives has been radically transformed. Despite all our superior medical technology, we have more deaths from COVID-19 than any other country. Why we do is the issue this book will explore.

The SARS-CoV-2 pandemic caught us unprepared and exposed our inability to respond medically and from a public health perspective. This inaction led to a profound health decline we haven't seen since the Second World War. What happened and why?

For an emergency physician presented with a sick patient, the first task is to consider that individual's vital signs. Those signs include the patient's pulse, blood pressure, and body temperature. We have a standard for an acceptable pulse and blood pressure. If the patient is stable and has a regular pulse between 45 and 100, there is no need to act immediately. Outside of that range, it may be necessary to intervene and fix that indicator. Similarly, for blood pressure and temperature, too high or too low is not good for remaining alive.

This book is about nations, however, not individuals. What are the vital signs for a country? And what are the acceptable values for those? I consider mortality measures to be the vital signs for a population. When I was a practicing emergency physician, the easiest diagnosis I could make in the emergency department was that someone was dead. All I had left to do was fill out a death certificate. When focusing not on an individual, but a nation, who is alive and who died in any given year is the most vital of the signs to assess that nation's health. How many are dying and how many are living? What are their ages? Their genders? Their socioeconomic status? Where do they live? How do they live? How has COVID-19 affected those national vital signs?

Many nonfiction books written for popular audiences, especially those dealing with health topics, begin with a personal story. Uncle Joe with diabetes. Or Blind Willie Johnson and his difficult life. Consider Aunt Emma, who died alone in the hospital from COVID-19.

DOI: 10.4324/9781003315889-1

If a story were to begin this book, it would be about the United States of America as the patient. We are not used to stories about countries, but are instead accustomed to stories about the people in those countries. We connect to tales of heroism through good character, risk-taking, and hard work. In contrast, when a character suffers misfortune, they are often presented as failing due to their weak temperament, bad decisions, or laziness. In a country founded on the myth of meritocracy, success is viewed as a personal achievement and failure as the result of individual failings.

Once we focus on the individual's story, however, it becomes impossible to look beyond that narrative to know how that same problem is experienced by an entire nation. A nation's problems come from collective decisions made by its people, as well as those having considerable political and economic power, and are impacted by what other countries face and how they respond. Some nations do better than others in almost any circumstance, yet it might surprise some readers to learn how poorly the United States has done in a range of vital markers.

The challenge of *Inequality Kills Us All* is to get the reader thinking about the country as the patient, as the protagonist, and as the collectivity of its peoples' health and economic problems, instead of considering any single individual's problems and their potential solutions.

Every problem is there to teach you something. If you don't learn from it, there will be another similar one in the future to provide you a fresh opportunity. What is the lesson Americans[1] have to learn from COVID to avoid future tragic disruptions? To begin with, we neglected strong repeated warning signals regarding our health, signals showing that our health was deteriorating. We did not have proper safeguards in place to protect our health and well-being but focused on policies that distracted us from our problems. Our institutions, put in place to keep us healthy, failed the country. Reflect on that concept: Our institutions failed us. It was not because of a few bad apples that mortality rose in our patient, America. It was the whole barrel of apples that were rotten.

Other countries have been spared such a severe fate. Something is different in their values, culture, and political structure that has prevented such havoc. We have been the victims of believing in American exceptionalism, namely, that we know what is right and lead other nations. They learn from us. Yet, our COVID carnage and response demonstrate we have much to learn from other nation states. We are a sick society.

A sage once said not everything that can be counted counts. We can all agree that being alive counts. Mortality statistics count deaths and arrange them in various categories. How many died in their first year of life? That's infant mortality. How many died in the first five years of life? That's child mortality. How many died in adolescence? Adulthood? Old age? All you need to know to assess the health of a country's people is when someone began life, their birth-day, and when that person dies, their date of death. All rich countries record these events called vital statistics. The National Center for Health Statistics, a branch within our federal government, does this. Once we know this information about a given population, we can then calculate average length of life, which is the life expectancy or estimated life span of the people within that population. These are vital signs for a population, a country, or a part of a country, such as a state or a county.

Other vital measures that could be considered include indicators of wealth, poverty, environmental factors (such as, CO_2 emissions, air pollution, forest cover, and water availability and quality), social and financial support, homicides, imprisonment, opioid consumption, teen births, obesity, educational performance, and mental health, among many others. Since most of us prefer to be alive rather than dead, our choice of vital signs, our mortality rates, are critical for discussion and analysis.

What then are normal vital signs, or vital statistics, for a country? Consider infant mortality, the proportion of babies born who die in their first year of life. Infant mortality ranges from about 1.5 deaths per thousand live births to over 100 deaths according to our Central Intelligence Agency[2]. That is the range of infant mortality rates globally. But what rate is normal? There is no definition for normal infant mortality as there is for an individual's blood pressure or temperature. There is no number, as there is for a person, that requires us to act quickly to save lives. Fortunately, looking at other countries helps resolve this ambiguity.

What is the range for infant deaths throughout the world? In Afghanistan, one death occurs in every ten babies born in a year. A ten percent mortality rate is definitely not normal. Less than one infant death in 500 is much better and found in many countries—but not in the United States. I suggest that action should be required if the infant mortality rate becomes much different from that number. There is no reason why the best health indicator in the world shouldn't be the one considered normal. How does the U.S. rank for infant deaths? Despite bragging about having the best healthcare in the world, there is one infant death for every 175 babies born in America. Some fifty nations have lower infant death rates. Those with fewer infant deaths include all the other rich countries plus some that would surprise you such as Belarus, Slovenia, Cuba, French Polynesia, and Latvia.

How about women dying in childbirth? Using the same CIA website, we can come up with a normal maternal mortality ratio (the number of women who die of childbirth-related causes for every hundred thousand births). The lowest ratio is 2 deaths of mothers for every 100,000 babies born, common to quite a few nations, while the U.S. number is 19. Again, 55 countries have a lower chance of women dying from childbirth-rated causes than America.

The same is true for life expectancy, or average length of life, for a particular year. There are 46 nations where people enjoy a longer life than we do in the USA—and this is the statistic for 2019 before factoring in COVID-19's impact which reduced our country's life expectancy by over 2 years. Many other nations did not see a decline in life expectancy with COVID.

CIA rankings presented here come from our own government. The United Nations, the World Bank, the World Health Organization, and others report similar findings. No matter where we look, when considering mortality as our measure of health, and the ranges of normal vital signs for a country as I have discussed, American health is not normal. We are not healthy at least in terms of the proportion of us being alive at any time compared to many other nations.

Your response may be that those figures don't apply to me. You might think, I feel healthy, practice good health behaviors, and see my doctor. You can't tell me that just because I live in the greatest country in the world that there is something wrong with my health! Therein lies this book's challenge.

Prior to COVID-19, our health as people in the richest and most powerful nation in world history was not even close to the best possible health status. COVID-19 has wrought to America the most cases and deaths of any country. To be fair, if we report cases or deaths in proportion to the population size, we are not the worst, but we are in the top ten or twenty. Given that we didn't have good health to begin with, that shouldn't be a big surprise though it is still shocking. One reason it is shocking is because neither our poor health status nor our COVID-19 ranking usually appears in the news and various media that capture our attention.

Inequality Kills Us All will explore these details and present the reasons why we are dead first, namely, dying younger at pretty well all stages of life, compared to people in so many other nations. We do not have normal vital signs. Abnormal should not be our normal.

Chapter 1 details how the United States does in dealing with so many more deaths than other countries. In the early 1950s, we had some of the best health outcomes, measured by death rates, of any country. Health has improved considerably since then but health, measured by death rates, improved faster in many other nations than in the United States. In those 70 years, we went from being among the healthiest nations, to falling behind all the other rich nations in mortality measures. A substantial number of middle and low-income countries have surpassed us too. Recently, we have seen increased death rates this century. We are not only not improving but also becoming worse. When vital signs of a nation deteriorate, when death rates go up, we have a serious emergency to deal with. But we haven't been paying attention nor keeping our eyes on our nation's health scorecard. COVID-19 sounded the call to action. Was our failing response caused by our vastly rising economic inequality? Or does it have something to do with how we raise children? Or was it our healthcare?

Chapter 2 considers the impact of healthcare on health. The most difficult issue for Americans to face requires recognizing the limitations of healthcare to produce health. Most of us conflate the terms health and healthcare when we speak of "accessing health," "paying for health," "getting health," and "insuring health." All those statements refer not to health itself, but to *healthcare*. Do we want health or healthcare? Ideally, we should have both, but we don't enjoy either in this country. COVID-19 attests to the imperfect medical care system we have as many died needlessly. Most expert analyses, including that by our government, do not attribute much health production through consuming medical or healthcare. What matters then?

Chapter 3 presents the studies that link economic inequality, whether income or education or other measures of social hierarchy, to health outcomes. Inequality, a comparative measure, is a property of a society, not an individual. This concept fits with our population health perspective. More income inequality causes worse health outcomes. A large income or wealth gap between the rich and the rest of us is toxic to society. While many politicians and analysts now voice this poisonous concern, most do not speak of inequality's detrimental impact on our health. But population health scholars are adamant. Inequality kills. It kills by increasing deaths at younger ages from most of the illnesses and diseases we face as we get older. This inequality that leads to early death is a form of structural violence or social murder. Inequality causes more deaths than the behavioral violence that we see and fear on the nightly news. Inequality kills many more people than gunshot wounds, car crashes, and drug overdoses—although inequality also plays a role in those deaths. COVID-19's lesson is that there is no smoking gun. Just like the coronavirus, there is no visible killer. Inequality has soared with SARS-CoV-2. Pandemic profiteering compounds the carnage as poverty increases.

Chapter 4 considers poverty as inequality's sibling. They live together. Being poor is bad for your health; it shortens your life. Yet, poverty is a recent human invention along with agriculture. Now global, various countries deal with poverty differently. In the United States, we tend to blame the poor for their outcomes. They represent personal failures. Other nations consider poverty a disability and provide safety nets. As poverty rises, so does inequality, and in this book, we ask, when does inequality impact health the most?

Chapter 5 shows that early life is the effector arm of inequality, the period when economic inequity has its greatest impact. In this country, we focus on end of life care, rather than nurturing early life. About half of our health is programmed between conception and age two. These first thousand days matter most for adult health. Societies can choose between early life or early death through policies that support the early years as well as old age. The nation can provide a relatively hazard-free period for the first thousand days of an infant's life by having, for example, a national policy of paid parental leave. Only two nations globally do not have such a policy—Papua New Guinea and the United States. Not only does the lack of such a policy compromise early life, COVID-19 has further jeopardized early life here. The failure to provide paid parental leave will lead to poor health in the adults these infants become. The United States doesn't invest in early life where the greatest return lies. Instead, the country pays for remedial actions to repair broken men and women, especially those over age 65. Our priorities are misplaced, in large part through lack of knowledge about what happens to adult health early on in life.

Chapter 6 exposes that certain groups within a nation have worse health through no fault of their own. Health inequities are the unfair health outcomes that poorer people face. COVID-19 has brought this fact into stark reality with death rates being much higher among people of color and other marginalized groups. Those lower down the socioeconomic ladder have worse health outcomes. Health is transferred from one generation to the next. Slaves had poor health, and so do descendants of slaves, and the cycle keeps repeating. American Indians bore the brunt of American expansion and aggression, and Indigenous Americans continue to have the highest U.S. death rates. These outcomes were beyond individual control but result from a historical legacy. Health is political, meaning it depends on how power relationships are structured. How does this happen?

Chapter 7 looks at the biological underpinnings of early life, inequality, and the various forms of societal stress we encounter. We look at populations, nations, and subgroups within nations. But we begin by considering individuals with cells and organs whose biology, the way they function, is well understood. Economic inequality produces stress which impacts people through harming their cells and organs. The United States has among the highest stress levels in the world. Such pressure severely impacts our bodies and is especially toxic in early life. No pill or procedure can later remove the stressful effects of early life. Stress leads to inflammation in later life, which causes the various chronic illnesses we suffer and die from. How might we integrate all these concepts?

Chapter 8 outlines the political choices that a nation's citizens make that determine its hierarchy, namely, who gets what benefits and where those advantages come from. How much of a country's national income is commandeered by the government and how that revenue is allocated determines the health outcomes of that nation. Social spending is what a country spends on its inhabitants. This outlay can go to subsidize privilege by not taxing multi-millionaires or to provide social and economic benefits for children and families. Healthier European nations provided ongoing economic support for their citizens during the economic COVID crisis. In contrast, the United States has given its citizens just a few sporadic tax credits, while subsidizing the already wealthy to a greater degree than ever before. We must look to political action by Americans that will transform our health status into being one of the healthiest nations. What must be done to get there?

Chapter 9 presents the prescription to become a healthy nation. First, we must acknowledge how well—or how poorly—we are doing. Then, we need to consider what we might learn about producing health from other nations. Finally, are we making progress? The United States can and should set a goal of becoming one of the healthiest nations on the planet. We have set goals and achieved them before. But to do so, a buy-in is required. We could then craft a strategic plan and monitor our progress. Specific policies are required to reduce our record economic inequality. Then, we can use those proceeds to invest in early life. We are fighting World War III against SARS-CoV-2 and future pandemics. Previous world wars required global cooperation, leadership, a strategy, and gauging progress. This one is no different. Where do you fit in?

Chapter 10 brings you, the reader, into the military force to fight the war. World War III—the war to achieve global health—requires cooperation and working together on many fronts. This war requires a citizen army. We must marshal many troops with their various skills into platoons to work together for victory. We must create a social movement. Many mass organizing tools exist today that were unthinkable a few decades ago. They are being used to both good and bad effect in dealing with our pandemic. It is up to us to mobilize for good health.

An afterword updates the COVID-19 situation.

We begin that effort by considering how the richest and most powerful nation in world history fares when it comes to our health. In the following chapters, I share that history, and my prescription for restoring our nation's health.

Notes

1. America and Americans will be occasionally (and incorrectly) used to connote the United States of America, which is about a third of the total land mass of North and South America. Its peoples number almost a billion with those in the United States comprising only a third.
2. Central Intelligence Agency World Rankings website.

Chapter 1

How Healthy Are We
in the United States

America is another name for opportunity.

Our whole history appears like a last effort of divine providence on behalf
of the human race.

Ralph Waldo Emerson

As a child growing up in Toronto, Canada, I was hooked on the American Dream.
I was profoundly affected by what was happening in the United States. While
there were Toronto TV stations, those from Buffalo, New York had more interesting content. I became fascinated by *Scientific American's* articles, and I paged
through catalogues of science materials from U.S. suppliers. Before I enrolled
in the mathematics and physics program at the University of Toronto, I was
immersed in publications from graduate schools at Harvard, Princeton, MIT,
Stanford, and Caltech trying to decide which one I should attend. I had two
goals: to cure cancer or harness fusion (the energy of the sun).

Upon arriving at Harvard University to study for my PhD in mathematics,
however, I was struck by the many contrasts with my native Canada. The best in
America was clearly better than the top in Canada. But the worst in the United
States was considerably below that in Canada. I hadn't really seen poor people
in Canada compared to what was readily apparent around Boston. Racism was
in my face. I would see more firearms in a few days than I had ever seen in
Canada. But I could buy more stuff at cheaper prices so maybe coming to the
United States was worth it. When my friends back home asked me what it was
like living here, I said the best here was better and the worst was worse than in
Canada. But the average in Canada was better than the average in the United
States. That view remains my perspective after so many years in the country that
I and so many people desire to live in. And now, after living in the United States
and working as an emergency physician for over 30 years, I'm an American.

For nearly five centuries, the land that became the United States of America
has been a magnet for people yearning for a better life. And for many of us,
America has made good on its promises. We are the richest country in the
world, with constitutionally guaranteed freedoms that many other nations do

DOI: 10.4324/9781003315889-2

not enjoy. Our shores are protected by the strongest military possible. We can boast of winning the most Olympic medals, securing the most Nobel Prizes, and housing the most billionaires in the world[1]. Given these and other achievements, many around the world would like to make this nation their home to live the American Dream.

The tendency to believe that determination and focused efforts will get us wherever we want to go is part of our history. For both native-born and immigrants, the American Dream is alive and well—the belief that anyone, regardless of what circumstances they were born into, can rise above the social status they were hatched into and become successful. Ours is the land of opportunity, and of individuals who overcome incredible obstacles to achieve fame, wealth, and even health. These goals are achieved through sacrifice, risk-taking, and hard work, and not by chance. Dreams, of course, are fantasies, whether happening in your sleep, a hallucination after taking some substance, or a daydream for something better than you have. Dreams can be bad too. We learned that lesson tragically in 2020 when the nightmare of a deadly pandemic became a harsh American reality with COVID-19, demonstrating our lack of cooperation to battle the SARS-CoV-2 virus.

Given these dreams and lessons learned, how do we assess America's success when it comes to our well-being? Among the more objective ways to examine a nation's well-being is by looking at the health of its people. Serious illness prevents us from being able to enjoy life, to look forward to the future, to follow our dreams and inclinations. Being well is essential if we are to make the most out of our years on this earth. The ability to enjoy life, appreciate liberty, and pursue happiness depends on it. If you are dead, you can't enjoy life, whether you died from COVID-19 or a heart attack, or from being a victim of a mass shooting. With mortality or well-being as our measure, it may surprise many to learn that Americans do not enjoy the best health among nations. To better understand why this is, and what we can do about it, in this book, we'll explore and expose why we have such high mortality rates and low measures of well-being. We must reflect on the ways in which the wealthiest and most powerful country in world history has failed to produce good health among its citizens.

Life is just lessons. If we don't learn the lesson presented by COVID-19, we will have other opportunities to discover what we should have figured out previously. Those future encounters may be worse than what we are living through now.

Vital Signs and Vital Statistics: How Healthy Is America?

Vital is the key term here, relating to the seat of life. First, consider vital signs which are a marker of someone's general physical condition. Typically, when a patient came to the emergency department, the nurse would tell me that person's vital signs, measured soon after arrival as an indicator of how alive they were.

Temperature, pulse, breathing rate, and blood pressure were the critical numbers that gave me a sense of how quickly I had to act. If the person was resting comfortably with a pulse of 70, blood pressure of 120/80, a respiratory rate of 15, and a temperature of 98.6°F (37°C being the equivalent in almost every other nation), I could take my time. If the person was not arousable, had cold clammy skin, a pulse of 150, a respiratory rate of 30, and a blood pressure of 60/40, I'd be there in a heartbeat. With such parameters, blood, carrying oxygen and glucose (the form of energy in the blood), is not flowing adequately to sustain life. Such abnormal vital signs indicate death could be near so I had to act quickly. We know the range for normal vital signs, (the limits outside of which cause concern) for an individual person. What we need to do for our society, however, is to consider vital statistics as the vital signs of a nation.

Two vital markers in anyone's life are the most important for considering health. The first is when you were born, and the second is when you die. In the emergency department, the easiest diagnosis I could make was that someone was dead. Death is very hard to fake. In such a situation, I would fill out a death certificate, entering identifying details, date of death, and probable cause. The state in which I worked would collect these documents and link them to birth certificates.

With those data, knowing when someone was born and when they died, myriad mortality statistics can be computed. Infant mortality tabulates how many die in their first year of life, expressed as a proportion of births. Child mortality is when death occurs in the first five years. Adolescent mortality is if death occurs between age 10 and 19 years. Adult mortality is typically dying between age 15 and 60 years. Maternal mortality refers to when women die of childbirth-related causes. You can pick any age range to describe mortality rates. By integrating all these vital statistics for a country, you can calculate the average length of life in a given year if the mortality rates stayed the same. That is life expectancy, which is an important measure of the health of a society.

We will mostly not be looking at specific diseases and the mortality due to them. The cause of death I had to enter on the death certificate was often obscure—I could not always be sure of the exact cause of death. Of course, cardiac arrest, the heart stopping, is the ultimate cause for everyone. But what made that happen? Once we start considering diseases, then the response is typically disease-oriented. How do we cure a specific disease, limit its effects, or prevent it? We want to consider health in a broader sense than whether a specific disease is present or not. By doing so, we will discover a prescription for improving overall health rather than treating a disease. How might we apply that same thinking about what we need as individuals to remain healthy, to what we need as a nation to have a healthy population?

Such vital statistics are kept by all rich countries as well as many of those that are not so rich. In others, there are clever ways to estimate these indicators through surveys and demographic data. The sources of these vital statistics include our National Center for Vital Statistics, a branch of the federal

Department of Health and Human Services and similar organizations in other nations. You can find them for countries tabulated by the United Nations (UN), the World Health Organization (WHO), the World Bank, as well as our Central Intelligence Agency. "Our World in Data" is one trusted web-based resource from Oxford University that presents many indicators by country and over time. This information is available to anyone with internet access. The values of various mortality indicators we consider in this book don't differ much among the many sources above. What can we learn from exploring vital statistics as indicators of the health of a nation?

Let's start at the beginning, infant mortality. How many babies born in a given country die in the first year of life?

What is a normal infant mortality rate? The lowest is around two deaths per thousand births in 2019, as found in Japan and Iceland. The highest is over 100, as in Afghanistan. This is reported per thousand births for each year. The U.S. figure is 5.6, meaning out of every ten thousand babies born 56 will die in their first year (notice I multiplied by ten so we didn't have a fraction of a baby die). All the other rich nations, and a number of not-so-rich ones, have lower infant death rates than the United States(1). Despite having the perception that this nation has the most advanced medical knowledge and technology in the world, some 50 countries have fewer infant deaths than we do. This is not normal!

The astute reader may ask if those numbers are really comparable. After all, what is a live birth? Does a child who is born alive but dies within the first hours of its life count as a statistic for infant mortality? Does the definition of live birth vary in different countries? Yes, it does, but careful scrutiny shows the different definition of a live birth in France or the United States doesn't change the numbers or relative ranking much.

Since leaving my career as an emergency physician, I've been teaching at the University of Washington. In an effort to get my students thinking about health beyond the individual patient, I ask them to do a calculation based on comparing mortality indicators among different countries. I typically do this with child mortality, how many children die in their first five of life. I ask them to compare Slovenia and the United States and come up with how many fewer children would die every day in the United States if we had Slovenia's child mortality rate. They look up the data and perform a simple computation to discover that about 50 children die here *every day* who wouldn't die if we had Slovenia's rate. This number is considerably higher than mass shooting deaths, yet where is the alarm, despite these extra 50 children dying every day? Our children should not have to suffer this. Suppose you were one of those 50 families? I can say from personal experience that when my 4-year-old brother died, it was a great family tragedy that my parents constantly grieved for while I was growing up.

We can go through the list of many other mortality rates comparing countries and find similar results. Around 50 nations have lower death rates for the most commonly used indicators. To avoid drowning the reader in too many vital statistics, however, let's consider one other—how long we live—our life expectancy.

Average length of life, life span, and life expectancy are similar concepts that aggregate mortality for each age range and tally them up to give a single number. For the United States in 2019—before the pandemic—it was 78.9 years(2). That means if the death rates stayed the same for the next hundred years, someone born in 2019 could expect to live almost 79 years. Expect, here, is a technical term meaning expectation of life at birth. It doesn't mean that everyone will live that long and then just drop dead. Some will die in infancy and some will live to be a hundred. Seventy-nine years is the average length of life here. Given that statistic, our longevity looks pretty good. But how do other countries do?

To answer that question, we must consider which countries to look at. Only those that belong to the UN? Should we include countries with very small populations such as the Vatican, Monaco, and Martinique? For over 20 years, I've used UN data as the source recognizing that it does not include these tiny nations, nor Taiwan, and has the fewest countries of all agencies mentioned above. What we find when we look at that solid data is that in 2019, the UN has the United States showing a lower life expectancy than 35 other nations(2). The top 40 nations' life expectancy is graphed below. This is as good as it gets since every other source listed above puts us below even more countries because they include more tiny nations.

Over 20 years ago, I coined the term "Health Olympics" as a way of ranking countries by mortality and other indicators of health. Since countries compete in the Olympic games, it would be revealing to add health events to the competitions. Some might argue that those competing in the Olympics are individuals and teams. So, to be fair, we should choose our healthiest individuals to compete against similarly healthy contestants in other countries.

If we take our longest-lived state, Hawai'i, and compare it to life expectancy in other countries, people in some 25 nations have longer lives (Figure 1.1). What about our "oldest old" people, those who have lived for a century or more, the oldest person alive at any one time? Sorry, they are almost never found in the United States. By any measure you can construct, we are not among the finalists in health competitions.

I began tracking the United States standing in the Health Olympics beginning in the 1950s when we were in the top 10. When I went to medical school in 1970, we stood 17th. In 1992, when I entered public health school, we were 22nd. I felt confident then that America would not drop much further. And when we dropped to about 25th, in the late 1990s, I predicted we had bottomed out. I just couldn't imagine we wouldn't drop further. How wrong I was!

COVID has made the American situation considerably worse with some 50 countries having longer lives(3, 4). For 2020, the U.S. life expectancy has dropped to 77.3 years, or 1.6 years lower than in 2019(5). Our standing in the 2020 Health Olympics awaits the UN report. We will likely be around

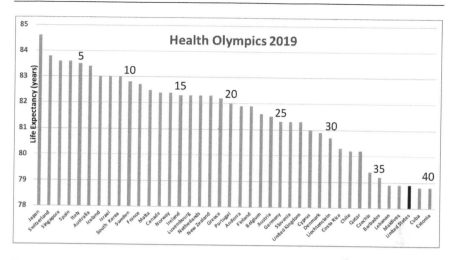

Figure 1.1 Ranking of the top 40 countries by life expectancy in 2019. Author's calculations from (2).

the 50th. For 2021, our rank appears to be below 60, meaning some 60 nations have longer life expectancies(6). That rank is due to our failure as a nation to respond effectively to the COVID-19 pandemic, leaving us as the nation with a high level of deaths per capita from COVID-19. It may be even worse, when we consider whether an older population affects life expectancy calculations and skews the results upward.

Many mortality measures depend on the age structure of the population. However, life expectancy calculations do not depend on whether there are many older people such as in Florida, where retirees settle, or a more youthful population as in Utah. Deaths toward the end of life impact the calculation of life expectancy less than deaths at younger ages. But again, what is the normal life expectancy?

Japan's life expectancy in 2019 was 84.6, or 5.7 years more than the United States and for 2020 the difference rose to 7.1 years! What is the significance of that difference? How can we operationalize that difference?

Our two leading killers are heart attacks and cancer. In 2019, they caused over 1.2 million deaths, or almost half of all the U.S. deaths. Suppose we eliminated those killers, cured heart disease and cancer, so no one died from them but left the other diseases to dispatch us to our graves. We would gain about 5.7 years of life expectancy according to a study by our National Center for Vital Statistics(7). For 2020, add in COVID-19 deaths and it doesn't speak well for health in America.

This points out how small differences in life expectancy among countries represent large differences in health outcomes. When I speak about this topic to various audiences and sense profound disbelief, I tell them to not believe a word that I have said. I ask them, if their health is important to them, that they verify what I have presented. For anything important to you, you shouldn't believe others. You must think critically, look at the data yourself, and come to your own conclusions.

Most younger readers of this book, don't think about the end of life and living to 80 years. Having a heart attack or cancer is not on their Instagram screen. They are in the moment here and now. You've survived infancy and childhood where our mortality is higher, but after is easy street and we need not to worry about dying young in comparison to other nations. Let's take 20- to 24-year-olds. Surely their chance of dying is not much different than that in other rich countries. If we compare the chance of dying in that age range to that of youth in Denmark or Spain in 2018, it is over four times higher. Unintentional injuries and homicide are the likely paths you will take to an early grave(8). And yes, young men have more than twice the chance of dying than women. As we will see in Chapter 6, the risk is greater in certain parts of the country, but nowhere is it safe enough. And if you think this doesn't apply to you because you do all the right health behaviors, Chapter 4 will show that to not be so.

To summarize these mortality data, we are dead first among many nations, including all the rich nations and a number of poorer ones such as Chile, Costa Rica, and Slovenia. That is, we do not enjoy longer lives if the standard is comparing ourselves to other nations. This book explores why this is the case and what "medicine" we need to be healthier.

Recall that we have figures for judging whether someone's vital signs are normal or not. "Normal" vital signs (or statistics) for a nation should be those indicating the best health. By these criteria, we in the United States do not achieve the normal health found in other countries. Why?

This may be the most health-conscious time in the U.S. history. We're bombarded with advice on what to do to be healthy. Get this Fitbit, eat this food, wear a mask, sanitize your hands, get immunized, don't smoke, watch your weight, drink coffee, don't drink coffee. Which new study should we prioritize? What will give each of us the best chance of living longer, staying free of deadly diseases like COVID-19, cancer, and diabetes, or dying of a stroke? These are questions that plague many of us, at least those with the time to be concerned after meeting the necessities of life—work, family caregiving, buying groceries, and paying the rent.

Besides being the richest country in world history, the United States is the global leader in science and technology and is supposed to have the best healthcare of any nation on earth. Why, then, does the U.S. rank among the worst of industrialized countries in chronic disease (diabetes, hypertension, lung disease), early death, infant and maternal mortality, suicide, and deaths from firearms? The answers often provided suggest that reversing these health threats is up to the individual—if we eat healthier foods, exercise more, seek preventative healthcare, and lock up our guns—we won't be among the tragic statistics that have plunged America into the dubious distinction of being the sickest industrialized nation on earth. But is it really just a matter of changing how you behave that will ensure you live a healthy life? Is our failure to provide universal healthcare the only obstacle to becoming the healthiest nation? And is it too late to reverse the trend the United States is headed toward as good health is increasingly a luxury few in the United States can enjoy?

Wait! I know that you, the reader, are not one of those eating junk foods, and only getting off the couch when the batteries in the remote control need to be replaced. Some of you may have a well-paying job, own your own house, can afford a vacation, and maybe even send your kids to private schools. Your neighbors are friends. You shop for organic foods, have a gym membership and go regularly. You might have a personal trainer. You may pay extra for a concierge doctor who you can call on her mobile phone at any time. So while you've seen those statistics about America's health being not up to the standard of other nations, this information doesn't apply to you. That other Americans don't have good health is their problem, not yours. But as you'll soon see, this book turns these ideas upside down.

The process of getting you to consider changing your deeply held beliefs is challenging. How do you come to know something is true? I ask this question when speaking to a variety of different audiences. I was once giving a talk in a grade 8 class in a private school near Seattle where some of the richest people in the world send their children. I was talking about how healthy we in the United States were and the reasons why. The students looked bewildered and were not allowed to distract themselves with their devices. I stopped and asked, "How do you know something is true?" Nobody answered. Uncomfortable silence followed. Rather than break the silence by saying something, I remained mute. Finally, one boy raised his hand and said, "If our parents tell us when we are very young, if our friends and teachers reinforce this idea, and if we have experienced it, then we know it to be true."

Epistemology is the branch of philosophy that asks how we know something to be so. It is the theory of knowledge or the investigation of what distinguishes justified belief from opinion. This boy was a stellar epistemologist. I've never found a more succinct explanation for deciding if a belief is true.

The world has changed considerably since that boy's conceptualization of truth. We are in the era of misinformation, disinformation, deep fakes, social turmoil, and political tribalism. How did such changes happen so quickly? We will argue later that those who are advantaged by the way things are today are continually at work to make us understand that this is the way they should be. Our commonsense view of the world should support those with power keeping it and have the rest of us being satisfied with less. After recognizing the political nature of health, we will come to see how our judgment has been polluted by some forms of social media in wicked ways that we explore in Chapter 9.

Our parents don't tell us what I've just said about American health, nor do our friends or teachers, and unless we look at mortality data, we can't experience the killer facts presented here to know whether they are true.

Ideas or concepts that we are exposed to in early life stay with us almost forever. Besides those thoughts, other factors in our development during this early period determine so many outcomes as we enter adulthood, as we age, and as we say goodbye to this life.

How do you experience health? I will share personal health and illness experiences throughout my life and muse on how they have shaped my views. Others have very different experiences of health and illness. Is there a way we can integrate these myriad circumstances and come to a common understanding?

Recall the grade 8 student's last point. "If we experienced it then we know it to be true." How do we experience or personalize mortality statistics? Consider it the biggest challenge we have in reconciling our preconceived views of health in America, with the harsh reality I'm presenting to you.

There are many personal and universal paths to pursue mortality here. In 1624, John Donne wrote his poem: "No man is an island." The poem ends:

> *Any man's death diminishes me,*
> *because I am involved in mankind;*
> *and therefore never send to know for whom the bell tolls;*
> *it tolls for thee.*

To understand our own health, we must accept, as Donne did almost 400 years ago, that the lives of others affect us. When older relatives of a child die, the child may understandably experience deep sadness. Grieving the deaths of parents, grandparents, and other elderly relatives is an expected part of life. The shock of the death of a peer, however, can provoke a surprisingly strong reaction as well. When I was in middle school, a classmate died from cancer. He and I had shared many common interests in science and life through vigorous discussions. The shock and fear of seeing someone my own age die made me so violently ill that I couldn't attend his funeral. Donne's universal had become personal. While I tend to forget many unpleasantries, I cannot obliterate this event from my memory.

We know we're impacted by the health of those important to us, but it turns out that the health of those we don't know affects our health as well. A key argument presented in this book is that failing to care for the health of others on a broad scale will ultimately compromise our own health. We will look at the health of people in various countries and begin to explore for whom the bell tolls.

But has it always been like this in America? Have we always had less than the best health? A look at our history reveals the answer.

History of Health in America

In the early 1950s, the United States had among the best health of all nations, measured by mortality indicators(9). Our maternal mortality in 1953 was the lowest of all countries, according to the WHO(10). Fifteen years later, however, although our maternal morality had declined, it had improved less than in other nations, so we no longer enjoyed the best outcomes for our mothers. The same was true for infant mortality and life expectancy. We were near the top of the rankings for the Health Olympics in the early 1950s. But health, measured by mortality, advanced faster in other countries than it did in the United States. Slower progress here results from the system we have created.

Joseph Stalin, the brutal Russian dictator responsible for millions of deaths, is reputed to have said, "The death of one man is a tragedy. A million deaths is just a statistic." Stalin, however, did put in place remarkable mechanisms to improve health in Russia despite arranging for killing millions during his reign. Statistics have a dehumanizing effect on the information being presented—it's much easier to empathize with an individual than with a number. Is each of the infants and young children who die needlessly every day in the United States a tragedy? Or those succumbing to heart attacks? Or dying from a car crash? Or are all these lives lost just a statistic, a set of numbers? Helping people humanize the suffering that lies behind these numbers is one of the main challenges of a "population health" approach. Mainstream media typically present health issues as stories or case histories of individuals; we tend to relate to the people they describe and their individual struggles. But it's important to also understand the larger context, the country, in which their stories take place.

The data described here, which show the United States at a substantial health disadvantage, are extremely relevant to the well-being of this nation, but are largely unrecognized. A typical response when I speak to a wide range of groups—from healthcare workers to students to the homeless—is total incredulity. How can it be that our health is so much worse in the United States than in other countries? We are, after all, the richest and most powerful nation in world history. What are we doing wrong?

Many would assume that medical professionals, and those in training, would learn this information about the U.S. health during their education. Is it part of the medical school curricula? A study in 2002 asked U.S. medical students how the United States ranked in health, in terms of highest life expectancy and lowest infant mortality. Fully a third thought we had the best indicators in the world(11). I find similar results when I ask for a show of hands among professional medical groups including professors of medicine. True, the health of this nation may not be directly relevant to most medical encounters, but perhaps if doctors were more involved in supporting health, rather than just providing medical or surgical treatment for illness and injury, the relevance would be more clear. A movement to incorporate such education into medical training has started in other countries, but not much has happened here.

How many Americans are aware of our being dead first? There are almost no published studies, other than the one of medical students mentioned above. One study looked at public perceptions of spending on healthcare and its relation to life expectancy. Americans believe that advances in healthcare produce better health, as measured by longer life expectancy. Next in importance were lifestyle factors. Public health and attention to what we will call Social Determinants of Health in Chapter 6 are not perceived as important by the American public, at least prior to COVID. Qualitative surveys of primary healthcare workers as well as senior undergraduate students conducted by two of my graduate students have shown a little more awareness, but these represent very small numbers interviewed.

To summarize, we in the United States have higher rates of death pretty well throughout our life spans compared to many other countries(12). Even before COVID-19, our health had been declining absolutely. Yet Americans are mostly unaware of this crisis. Even the rare brief mention in the media of our life expectancy decline doesn't include an interpretation of what this means in the context of our health comparable to eradicating heart disease and cancer or other causes of death. That we are not as healthy as the best should be of major concern.

Why are we so unaware of this fundamental issue? I've long been trying to come to grips with this conundrum. Partly, it is our individualistic focus. Our nation was built on the foundation of freedom from tyranny—we fought for independence, and framed our nation around concepts of individual liberties and human rights. In doing so, we have to forget slavery and destroying the indigenous population residing here. Another dark side of our greatness is that, in doing so, our civic responsibilities took a backseat. Our sense of ourselves as members of a community was weakened. Now, centuries and the internet later, we tend to conceptualize our citizenship as exclusively based on our rights, not our responsibilities. It's all about me. I'm alive so these deadly facts aren't about yours truly. There is also the role of technology and our relationship to our environment in our cultural perceptions as we established our nation through agriculture. We'll explore agricultural reasons for our individualism in Chapter 8. My point is, like all countries, our culture shapes our perceptions of ourselves and of the world. And one way American culture has shaped our view is in how we perceive health statistics. Americans don't take national numbers seriously, partly because we treasure our privacy. We want to be in control of information such as our birthday and later when we die. Birth and death statistics, representing national surveillance by the government, invade that realm. Despite our increasingly interconnected world, many Americans are not interested in the world beyond their shores and don't want to compare their health with others. Many of us don't know where to place many countries on a map, even with internet access. I even see that among my college students!

Another reason we don't think of our nation's health in a global context is that the U.S. statistical agencies don't tend to make comparisons with other nations— we measure ourselves against ourselves, with no regard for other nations.

The nonprofit think tank the U.S. National Research Council is our most regarded group of experts whose members are among the most respected scientist-thinkers. They have produced several reports comparing the U.S.

health with other rich nations(13, 14). The 2013 comprehensive report pointed out that even the healthiest of us lag behind similar people in comparable countries. The bell tolls for you!

Healthy Life Expectancy

You might say, "I don't care how long I live, I just want to have a healthy life." Yet most of us, given the choice, would rather live a longer life than a shorter one. When you read obituaries, the age at death is always presented. It is important to us that our lives aren't cut short. But does a longer life mean relinquishing a healthy body as we age? Are countries where people live longer lives those where they have more healthy years?

Unequivocally yes! A measure called Healthy Life Expectancy looks at not just the years lived, but those in which people have good or "full" health. The indicator adjusts for years living with illness or disability. Calculations for Healthy Life Expectancy include estimates of the prevalence and severity of important diseases and disabilities, as well as how long they last and how much they limit good health. Unhealthy years are then subtracted from standard life expectancy figures that consider only deaths. The WHO reports healthy life expectancy for its member countries, indicating how many years a person can expect to live in full health(15).

So how does the U.S. rank in *healthy* life expectancy? For 2019, we had 66 healthy years with some 69 countries ahead of us and Japan leading the world with 74 healthy years. Does that mean another eight years of drooling in a nursing home? That depends on where you live. Our rank, the number of nations living healthier lives, is worse partly because of the greater number of countries in the WHO list. But we are a sick nation. Four years earlier in 2015, we had more healthy years, 67 of those years in good health. So the Japanese not only live longer than we do, they also have eight more years without serious disability and illness. And although healthy life expectancy is increasing in most countries, in the United States it has fallen, consistent with our life expectancy declines that will be described in greater detail later. Ah, Japan again. It must be all the sushi they eat.

I've hinted that personal behaviors are not the main factors producing better health. We can all agree that smoking cigarettes is not good for your health. Perhaps some readers smoke and have tried to quit. Out of all the countries in the Health Olympics list I described above, the 35 nations where people lived longer lives in 2019, which one has the lowest proportion of men smoking? The United States and Sweden have about 15% of men smoking. Over twice as many men per capita smoke in Japan, and they have among the highest smoking rates in that list.

I first discovered this paradox over 20 years ago. This made me question the importance of health-related behaviors for producing health. My experience visiting in Japan verified that many men smoke there. In crowded cities, they have signs warning people not to smoke outside. That is to avoid cigarettes burning the eyes of children who may be walking behind you as you lower your lit cigarette after inhaling. If you've been at Narita Airport outside Tokyo, you may have passed by one of the many smoking rooms inside that are full of Japanese men puffing away. At the U.S. airports, there are only a few places, strategically placed outside, where people can smoke.

We can similarly discount dietary factors as the cause. Okinawa used to be the healthiest prefecture in Japan and their diet was predominately pork fat and noodles. I had read this before visiting Okinawa but was still surprised to see many slabs of pork fat in the markets along with cans of Spam, which is a staple there. How do they get away with eating stuff we can't imagine being good for health? *Hara Hachi Bu*—a Confucian teaching, instructing people to stop eating when they are 80% full—certainly helps.

This is not to say that personal behaviors don't matter for producing health. They are just overshadowed by other factors that this book exposes.

For the U.S. reader, consider that because you live in the United States, your health isn't as good as it could be if you were conceived, born, and grew up to live in quite a few other countries. Personal health-related behaviors, while important, are not as important as you think. Being rich in America is better than being poor here, but being of lower means in a number of other nations will give you better health than being well-off here.

What about Happiness?

Is living in "full health," as indicated in the Healthy Life Expectancy characterization, just a physical phenomenon? What about the feeling of well-being, a sense of general satisfaction with the state of one's life, the honest response to the social greeting, "How are you?" Recall that the U.S. Declaration of Independence entitles us to the right to life, liberty, and the pursuit of happiness. Although we have the right to life, it's clearly not a long life compared to people in other nations today. Are we successful in our pursuit, especially compared to those others?

Even though happiness is a much more subjective state than being alive or dead, the study of happiness and its production is well-established. Books for the lay reader tell us how to be happier, as well as how to be healthy, presenting individual perspectives that explain what you can do as an individual to lead a fulfilling life. But another perspective involves comparing happiness or quality of life among people in different countries and considering the societal or collective phenomena that make "happiness," however defined, more likely.

The Sustainable Development Solutions Network of the UN produces a yearly *World Happiness Report* from global surveys through Gallup World Polls. It asks the following question: "Please imagine a ladder, with steps numbered from 0 at the bottom to 10 at the top. The top of the ladder represents the best possible life for you, and the bottom of the ladder represents the worst possible life for you. On which step of the ladder would you say you personally feel you stand at this time?" Surveys are regularly carried out using this question with a representative population sample in some 150 countries. The results are people's evaluations of their overall quality of life—what we might call happiness.

In the 2021 report of the happiness indicator for the period 2018–20, the United States came in at number 19, with the top three nations being Finland, Denmark, and Switzerland(16). That report was especially concerned with COVID-19 in various parts of the world. Previous reports reported changes in happiness such as in the period 2008–12 compared to 2017–19 which was presented in the 2020 report when the U.S. happiness indicator declined significantly. During that period gains were registered in over 60 nations. Many other sources show happiness declines in the United States. Surveys of students in the classes I teach on population health respond that they believe happiness is declining here. Readers are likely to at least consider that our right to pursue happiness has not succeeded.

Changes in happiness over this period were tallied from those nations registering gains in happiness and those with declines. Out of the 149 countries presented in the 2020 report, the United States ranked 113th from the top for changes in happiness. Our happiness declined from 2008–12 to 2017–19(17). Only 36 nations had worse declines in happiness than the United States in that report. These nations include Brazil, India, and Libya. While we are pursuing happiness with a vengeance that happy state is eluding us more and more.

Chapter 7 in the 2020 report is entitled, "The Nordic Exceptionalism: What Explains Why the Nordic Countries are Constantly Among the Happiest in the World?" Their conclusion speaks of institutional and cultural indicators that include a well-functioning democracy, social welfare benefits, low levels of crime, and corruption with the citizenry feeling free and trusting of both each other and governmental institutions. Similar ideas in previous *World Happiness Reports* as to why the US is not doing well in happiness consider income inequality as a major explanation of our problems (the key point of Chapter 3).

Other studies on well-being and happiness use somewhat different measures, but the United States fails to reach the top ten in any of them. In many surveys, well-being in the United States shows a steeper decline for women than for men. The quality of our lives in the United States is not exemplary, but instead mirrors what we learn from studying deaths.

To summarize, whether we look at health by death rates or feeling satisfied with life, as a nation the United States does not do well. Renown epidemiologist Geoffrey Rose captured this point clearly in his book, *The Strategy of Preventive Medicine*, saying there is no biological reason why a population's health should not be at the level of the best possible(18). Countries with superior health statistics such as Japan demonstrate what is attainable. Improving the health and well-being of Americans is not a hypothetical paradise like Shangri-La, but rather something that has already been achieved elsewhere. And if America is still the land of opportunity, we can do it here.

Conclusion

Although we've been taught to believe America is the greatest nation on earth, when it comes to our health, we are far from the best. We have higher infant mortality, higher child and maternal mortality, live shorter lives, and suffer more chronic illnesses. This dire state has only worsened with COVID-19 which has disrupted most people's lives profoundly. The United States has had more cases and deaths from COVID-19 than any other country. Our public health system was not up to the challenge, so we paid the ultimate price. We are desperate to get back to normal, or at least to our pre-COVID state. In this chapter, we have seen that BC (before COVID-19) normal was pretty abnormal, at least in the United States. What are the lessons we must learn from the pandemic to have more healthy lives than we were living before we were invaded by SARS-CoV-2?

COVID-19 has made us grave diggers as we have faced our mortality. The pandemic has also diminished our well-being. Despite spending much more on healthcare than any other nation, American medical care has been pushed to its limits. Is it our healthcare system that we need to fix to accomplish this? Or might there be another answer?

Questions to Consider and Discuss

1. Why has there been so little discussion of the poor health status of Americans?
2. Happiness appears to be declining in the United States, with more among women than men. Is this consistent with your experiences? Why is this taking place?

Note

1. China may have surpassed the United States in terms of most billionaires during 2021.

References

1. Central Intelligence Agency. Country Comparison: Infant Mortality Rate Washington, D.C.: Central Intelligence Agency; 2021 [cited 2021 November 1]. Available from: https://www.cia.gov/the-world-factbook/field/infant-mortality-rate/country-comparison.
2. UNDP (United Nations Development Programme). Human Development Report 2020 The Next Frontier Human Development and the Anthropocene. New York, NY: United Nations Development Program; 2020.
3. Aburto JM, Schöley J, Kashnitsky I, Zhang L, Rahal C, Missov TI, et al. Quantifying Impacts of the COVID-19 Pandemic Through Life-Expectancy Losses: A Population-Level Study of 29 Countries. International Journal of Epidemiology. 2022;51(1):63–74.

4. Woolf SH, Masters RK, Aron LY. Effect of the Covid-19 Pandemic in 2020 on Life Expectancy Across Populations in the USA and Other High Income Countries: Simulations of Provisional Mortality Data. BMJ. 2021;373:n1343.

5. Ortaliza J, Ramirez G, Satheeskumar V, Amin K. How Does U.S. life expectancy compare to other countries?: Peterson-KFF Health System Tracker; 2021 [cited 2021 September 28]. Available from: https://www.healthsystemtracker.org/chart-collection/u-s-life-expectancy-compare-countries/#item-start.

6. Commonwealth Fund Commission on a National Public Health System. Meeting America's Public Health Challenge: Recommendations for Building a National Public Health System That Addresses Ongoing and Future Health Crises, Advances Equity, and Earns Trust. New York, NY: The Commonwealth Fund; 2022.

7. Arias E, Heron M, Tejada-Vera B. United States Life Tables Eliminating Certain Causes of Death, 1999-2001. National Vital Statistics Reports. 2013;61(9):1–128.

8. Rogers RG, Hummer RA, Lawrence EM, Davidson T, Fishman SH. Dying Young In The United States: What's Driving High Death Rates Among Americans Under Age 25 and What Can Be Done? Population Bulletin. 2022;76(2):1–31.

9. Kinsella K. Changes in Life Expectancy 1900-1990. Am J Clin Nutr. 1992;55(6): 1196S–202S.

10. World Health Organization. Maternal Mortality. World Health Statistics Report. 1969;22(6):335–6.

11. Agrawal JR, Huebner J, Hedgecock J, Sehgal AR, Jung P, Simon SR. Medical students' Knowledge of the U.S. Health Care System and Their Preferences for Curricular Change: A National Survey. Academic Medicine: Journal of the Association of American Medical Colleges. 2005;80(5):484–8.

12. Bezruchka S. The Hurrider I Go the Behinder I Get: The Deteriorating International Ranking of U.S. Health Status. Annual Review of Public Health. 2012;33(1):157–73.

13. Woolf SH, Aron L, editors. U.S. Health in International Perspective: Shorter Lives, Poorer Health. Washington, D.C.: The National Academies Press; 2013.

14. Crimmins EM, Preston SH, Cohen B, National Research Council. Explaining Divergent Levels of Longevity in High-Income Countries. Washington, D.C.: National Academies Press; 2011.

15. The Global Health Observatory. Healthy Life Expectancy (HALE) at Birth (Years) Geneva: World Health Organization; 2020 [cited 2020 December 4]. Available from: https://www.who.int/data/gho/data/indicators/indicator-details/GHO/gho-ghe-hale-healthy-life-expectancy-at-birth.

16. Helliwell JF, Layard R, Sachs J, De Neve J-E, Aknin LB, Wang S, editors. World Happiness Report 2021. New York, N.Y.: Sustainable Development Solutions Network; 2021.

17. Helliwell JF, Layard R, Sachs J, De Neve J-E, editors. World Happiness Report 2020. New York, N.Y.: Sustainable Development Solutions Network; 2020.

18. Rose GA. The Strategy of Preventive Medicine. New York, NY: Oxford University Press; 1992.

Chapter 2

Healthcare in America

primum non nocere[1]

My earliest memory as a child was lying in a hospital bed at the Hospital for Sick Children in Toronto. I had been hospitalized for an infection of some sort, perhaps polio, as this was at the height of the polio epidemic. My bed faced a tall window into a hospital courtyard. Once or twice a day, my mother and father would appear on the other side of the window to smile, wave, and then look forlornly at me. They stood on a ledge outside in the cold, as I was in isolation and they weren't allowed in.

Doctors became an important part of my life. When I was just 2 years old, my 4-year-old brother died tragically in my mother's arms after a short illness. This tragedy changed our family dynamic profoundly: my mother and father grieved over the loss for the rest of their lives. Our only family outing for many years was the weekly trip to the cemetery. They wouldn't risk losing another child—seeing the doctor when sick became a part of my life—they even made house calls throughout my childhood, something unheard of these days.

I revered doctors for being lifesavers. Medical care could really heal, and I wanted to become the medical hero my parents didn't have to save my brother. I wanted to cure others and to save lives. Dazzled by the magic of medical science, I just didn't understand the limitations of that knowledge.

Healing the Sick

That healthcare is the pathway to health is an implicit assumption for many. In the United States, we speak of insuring health, accessing health, and paying for health. These expressions might lead us to believe that it is healthcare (in whatever form) that produces health. In actuality, we insure healthcare, access healthcare, and pay for healthcare. Some of us even provide healthcare. But does that care make us healthy?

During a medical career spanning nearly four decades, my focus was on diagnosing and treating diseases and injuries. However, although it's increasingly recognized that producing health is far more complex than simply treating

DOI: 10.4324/9781003315889-3

injuries and illnesses, that concept has not yet had a noticeable impact on our healthcare system. Modern medical care continues to reliably diagnose and treat illness and injury. But does a *lack* of medical care *make us* sick or *cause* the injury in the first place? Of course not. Therein lies the fallacy of considering access to care as the key to better health.

Why the High Costs of the U.S. Healthcare?

The prominence of healthcare as a national concern in the United States is reflected by the money we spend on it: more than any other nation and, in fact, almost as much as the rest of the world combined. In 2019, we spent $3.8 trillion on healthcare, or almost $11,000 per person. This astronomical figure represents 18% or more than a sixth of our total economy. What do we get for this investment? Certainly not health; as you've learned, our health status lags behind that of some 50 other countries. We spend massive amounts on healthcare without any demonstrable benefit to the population's mortality or other health measures.

Before COVID-19 expenditures for 2020 were projected to rise to $4 trillion. But they suffered a slight decline partly due to fewer people going to hospitals, or doctors and not receiving dental care as a result of the pandemic. Whether the industry will make up lost growth remains to be seen.

Chasing profits in the healthcare industry is a significant factor in producing the high medical bills that Americans face. In theory, market competition should result in lower prices. Why has this not happened? One explanation is the inaccessibility of information regarding how much a service costs. Patients are unable to shop for affordable healthcare because they don't discover the price of their treatment until they receive a bill weeks or months later. We aren't conditioned to ask about the cost of a service when seeking medical care, unlike the practice for most other products and services we purchase.

Consider a procedure such as a colonoscopy performed in a specific hospital and how much the amount charged varies. In an investigation of medical costs, *The New York Times* found that the actual charge for one hospital varied tenfold depending on which healthcare insurance carrier was billed or whether the patient had healthcare insurance (if not, the cost can be higher than that charged to insurance companies)(1). A pregnancy test in one major hospital varied ninefold depending on insurance or private pay. Even within an insurance plan, the bill depends on particulars of the plan. In 2021, as these costs came to light, the federal government ordered hospitals to begin publishing their prices they negotiate with their private insurers, though most have been slow to do so and resist the order.

One result of this lack of transparency is that bills for medical care are typically inflated, much like the bright sticker prices on a new car which the dealer sets and often has little relation to the manufacturer's suggested retail price. Various medical care insurers pay a discounted portion of the sticker price, then you are billed for what remains. There are also inflated administrative costs, fraud, and prices for products and services beyond any competitive benchmarks. The uninsured in particular are left in helpless confusion. Yet you might be surprised to learn that it wasn't always like this.

I learned about these and similar practices firsthand in the late 1970s. My group of emergency doctors was the first in Seattle to bill for our services separately from the hospital invoice. After each patient left, I wrote down codes for services and calculated an amount for the fee. If the patient had few resources, the level of service was typically downgraded and a smaller charge generated. During my 30 years as an emergency doctor, I can recall only one person—a young child's father—asking about the fee before I treated his daughter when he came with her to the ER in Seattle. His family did missionary work in Africa and had limited resources, so I reduced his daughter's bill after he explained their constraints. But if you ask a healthcare worker today what their fee will be before receiving a service, the answer will almost certainly be, "I don't know." That's not a lie intended to mislead patients; the healthcare workers genuinely don't know.

Eventually, our group contracted for a service to calculate the billing for care received. The contract gave a percentage of the bill to the company, who hired coders—typically nurses—to create bills from medical records. They urged us to increase charges by creating a medical record that would allow higher bills to be generated. "Be paid what you are worth," they told us, a catchphrase that encouraged us to amp up our medical fees, while alleviating our conscience for doing so. "Listen to the patient's heart, do a more detailed physical exam, and we can charge for that, as well," we were told. At the time, the tactics were troubling. Now, decades later, such billing techniques are the norm throughout the country.

These billing schemes partially explain the ongoing increases in medical care costs. Electronic medical records (EMRs) have now supplanted the paper medical record and led to a bizarre situation where medical scribes—physicians' assistants and others—document the encounter between a doctor and the patient, entering the details in the EMR which the doctor then signs off. Many healthcare workers detest the way EMRs are set up which is to make it easier to bill more for medical services, rather than provide the information required to render good patient care which the old written records had done. Today there is essentially no connection between the person who provides services—usually a doctor, but often a nurse practitioner, physician's assistant, or another healthcare worker—and the calculation of the amount charged. Such a disconnection helps make medical care a huge growth industry in the United States.

Many Americans believe that the profits in healthcare lead to higher quality healthcare. In the 1980s, we were told that government was the problem and the private sector performed better. Yet studies show that for equally sick patients, being treated in for-profit hospitals carries a greater risk of dying than those treated in public hospitals.

The dialysis industry is a good example. Not-for-profit dialysis centers have been displaced by for-profit facilities in the United States over the last few decades. In 1973, the Social Security Act provided for coverage of end-stage kidney disease treatment costs by Medicare. The kidney has thus become the only federal organ in the body, meaning that anyone with kidney failure (except those undocumented) requiring dialysis will have the costs covered by Medicare, a federal government program. But that consumer protection—a guarantee that kidney disease will be treated regardless of ability to pay—has brought new opportunities for the private sector, seeking profits. With the corporatization of kidney dialysis, today two businesses now control 85% of the U.S. dialysis market. Both have higher rates of mortality than patients receiving dialysis in a nonprofit facility(2). U.S. death rates for dialysis patients are as much as three times higher than in other rich countries(3). Although having a kidney transplant would improve one's chances of having a longer, healthier life, patients are often provided dialysis services by these centers for years on end. As profit-making centers, if their patients sought kidney transplants, which would get them off dialysis, they would lose business. COVID provides another example of how healthcare profits affect our health.

When COVID-19 relief funds became available, they were rapidly scooped up by the large nonprofit hospitals and for-profit chains through FEMA and CARES[2] legislation. Though larger chains have substantial investment portfolios and rainy-day funds, their ample assets didn't stop many of them from receiving federal "relief." With the adverse publicity generated by these corporate opportunists, some such as the nonprofit Kaiser Permanente System and the for-profit Healthcare for America returned the CARES act relief saying they didn't need it. And while small community nonprofit hospitals have been hardest hit by COVID-19 expenses, as the funds were directed toward larger hospitals and medical chains, there has been less funding available for these smaller hospitals.

There are a variety of other ways to profit from healthcare, none of which aim to improve quality of services. Medical businesses may hire less-skilled workers, work them harder, and cut costs for equipment and facilities. Medical assistants are one example. The profession of medical assistants initially became a career path for Army medics after World War II, as "nursing" was still considered women's work, but "medical assistants" were perceived as quasi-physicians. As these (mostly men) became more ubiquitous in the medical field, they became viewed as affordable substitutes for physicians, thereby cutting costs to the healthcare provider. Because the objectives of for-profit healthcare institutions are to generate revenue, with providing healthcare the strategy toward that objective, cutting the costs of healthcare gains priority over providing the best healthcare. It's an unfortunate fact that profit-oriented care, as practiced by the medical industrial complex, is the foundation of our healthcare system, and nonprofit systems must compete on those same terms.

The lobbying sector is another force that strongly influences the high costs of medical care. Lobbyists represent pharmaceutical and healthcare organizations, including doctors, hospitals, nursing homes, services such as dialysis, and many other aspects of the delivery of healthcare. This industry is huge, spending more than three times as much as lobbyists for industries such as defense, for example. Over four billion dollars was spent on lobbying to organize fundraisers, provide other benefits for lawmakers and influence laws regarding pharmaceutical and other medical products in the last two decades, which is at least a billion dollars more than any other industry. When I describe the lobbying industry to international students and ask them what such practices would be called in their countries, the response is uniform: corruption. Yet lobbying is legal in the United States and is thus not considered corruption.

Another explanation for the high cost of U.S. medical care is the inefficiency built into our healthcare delivery systems, which results in immense administrative expenditures. A study in 2017 found almost 35% went to administration which was double that spent in Canada(4). Administrative costs also appear to be increasing faster than other expenditures for healthcare, such as for doctors' services.

One reason for high administrative costs relates to the multiplicity of the payers from private insurance companies to businesses and individuals, with their complex set of procedures for reimbursement. The healthcare insurance industry brings in particularly strong profits, estimated to be $100 billion in 2005, and certainly more today. Profits for the second quarter of 2020 were twice those in the same quarter of 2019. The first two quarters of 2021 have been even more profitable for the big insurers, in part because people have sought less medical care because of COVID-19 concerns while they still pay medical insurance premiums. Such pandemic profiteering makes it difficult to restrain the power of healthcare insurance companies, and the exploration of alternatives is essentially not allowed. Recall the extensive public debate about the Patient Protection and Affordable Care Act (PPACA, shortened to ACA and nicknamed Obamacare). The so-called public option could have resulted in massive cost savings, but was never even officially discussed. Healthcare insurance company profits remain astronomical, as evidenced by the stock market share prices which, for the biggest companies, have risen fivefold since the ACA began. While today there are attempts to dismantle the ACA altogether, discussions of the public option, single-payer and "Medicare for all" have at least entered the public realm.

Unlike most rich nations, the United States does not provide access to healthcare as a fundamental right. The 1948 United Nations Universal Declaration of Human Rights enshrined medical care as a human right. But some, promoting the repeal of the Affordable Care Act, argue that healthcare is not a right, but a privilege. But what does that privilege—or lack of it—mean to those it affects? People who can't afford needed healthcare are essentially marginalized and powerless. The privileged get unrestricted access. Nearly one in ten people in the United States in 2019 were uninsured, and a considerably larger number were substantially underinsured. The leading cause of bankruptcy in the United States is the inability to pay medical bills, even for an insured person! This fate is incomprehensible to those from other rich nations. But awareness of the injustice of viewing healthcare as a privilege is growing, the winds of change hopefully leading us toward developing a society in which everyone has access to necessary services.

Linking Healthcare to Health

When I was studying at Stanford Medical School, Dr. John Bunker, the chief of its Department of Anesthesiology, was interested in how medical care affected health. He later teamed up with Frederick Mosteller at Harvard and John Frazier at University College London to study the impact of medical care on health. Their analysis estimated how much of the 30-year gain in life expectancy in the United States during the last century could be explained by medical care(5). Clinical trials, the gold standard for researching the outcomes of treatment for a particular disease or problem, formed the basis of their study. In a clinical trial, one group gets a specific treatment, while the other receives a placebo (something mimicking the treatment but without any active ingredient or principle), allowing researchers to isolate the effect of the treatment through comparison of the two groups.

Their research concluded that 5 years of the 30-year gain in U.S. life expectancy during the last century could be attributed to curative and preventive medical care, with immunization against diphtheria and smallpox, one of the biggest factors, and treating heart disease by managing hypertension and implementing cardiac care units also significant. There were lesser, but still demonstrable, gains they ascribed to the treatment of diabetes, pneumonia, and many other illnesses. In total, about three and a half years' gain was attributed to curative services, and a year and a half to preventive care.

Experts point out that the most important factor in the large health improvements seen in the last 150 years is not so much related to medical care, but to better hygiene and higher standards of living(6). Sewage is separated from drinking water. We wash our hands, cover our mouths and noses when sneezing or coughing, and keep our food away from flies. With the rise of COVID-19, we also recognized the importance of physical distancing, wearing effective masks, not shaking hands, and other behaviors intended to mitigate the spread of contagion. Yet we continue to think that if we spend more on our healthcare, we can buy our way to health.

Consider what we spend and what health we get. Figure 2.1 shows trends in healthcare expenditure for ten industrialized countries for each year from 1995 to 2015, along with life expectancy trends for those years(7). The dollar amounts are adjusted for purchasing power, so each dollar has the same ability

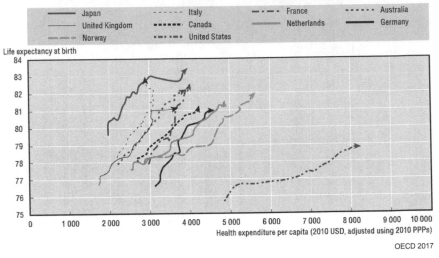

Figure 2.1 Healthcare expenditure and life expectancy trends from 1995 to 2015 for ten rich countries from (7).

to buy the same item in different countries. For example, Japan, with the solid line at the left, spent less than $2000 per person on healthcare in 1995 and their citizens had a life expectancy then of nearly 80 years.

The United States, the line at the lower right, is an outlier, spending the most by far, with the lowest life expectancies. By 2015, the United States hadn't attained Japan's 1995 life expectancy! All the other rich nations had lower costs and longer lives.

Whatever we are buying with our so-called health dollars is not health. Perhaps our way of organizing and providing healthcare is flawed. Or does healthcare have at best a limited impact on producing healthy societies? There is truth in both perspectives. Yet one paradox stands out. If spending so much on healthcare does so little to improve our health, why do we look to medical care with such reverence?

Medical Mediatization

When it comes to "health news," we don't learn about our nation's health. Instead, we are treated to stories designed to frighten us. Media coverage of the Ebola outbreak in Africa led to a phantom epidemic of anxiety in the United States yet more people died from HIV in a week than in the entire period of the Ebola outbreak. The H1N1, or swine flu, pandemic in 2008 caused considerable alarm. Frenzied Zika virus reports of disturbing images of birth defects shocked us. Along comes the SARS-CoV-2 epidemic. And the media have had a field day in presenting the horrors of COVID-19.

Patient heroism stories also abound. An individual's battle with cancer is a standard metaphor of stories of individual courage and determination—and success. Headlines such as "Tenacious 97-year-old WWII Veteran beats COVID-19" and a much younger person, "dies after battle with COVID-19" remind us of such bravery. The burden is on us to be courageous in our "fight" against death and disease. The media perpetuate such courage as they present those who survive as heroes, and those who don't survive as tragedies. Yet instead of beating the odds, we can lower the odds so that most of us will survive—but doing so won't necessarily make headlines.

Sensational new medical discoveries, new procedures, new diseases, and new drugs do make headlines. Take transcatheter aortic valve implantation, also known as TAVI. You can now be awake while a cardiologist inserts a collapsed heart valve made from a cow's outer heart lining into the space where the diseased heart valve sits. It is then inflated to take the place of the old valve. This is a remarkable technological breakthrough. Surgery can now be done on a fetus with a serious congenital heart disorder to repair the heart before birth. Stem cells are another newsworthy innovation. Given these amazing technologies, we've come to believe that there is no health problem medical care can't solve eventually.

Biomedicine has merged with the media to produce bio-mediatization. Media professionals work with healthcare leaders to co-produce programs to increase our understanding of healthcare and illness(8). Everyone can be considered an expert in biomedical knowledge, just by searching the internet. Devices and apps are designed to track our health as they monitor our exercise, diet, yoga routines, sleep, brain fitness, and much more. This resulting bio-mediatization machine, beholden to corporate and commercial interests, may not be good for our health.

Being an informed person on health matters is critical to navigating the highways and byways of the medical care industry. Yet for all the information now available to us, trying to separate fact from opinion, disinformation and misinformation, alternative facts, and justifiable conclusions has become extremely difficult but necessary.

Perhaps one of the biggest impacts media has had on how we think about our health and medical care has been through pharmaceutical ads suggesting you "ask your doctor" about prescribing whatever medicine they're pitching. When discussing whether these drug ads are a good idea, one of my students asked, "But without the ads, how will we know what drugs to ask for?" Forget the litany of required side effects paraded at the end of the ad which have become fodder for Saturday Night Live skits, but do little to discourage interest in the drugs, even when the side effects include sudden death. The ads are not otherwise regulated, and often contain much misleading content. Some of the drugs advertised are not only unnecessary, they may be harmful.

Only two countries—New Zealand and the United States—allow this kind of advertising to the general public. Why don't other nations follow America's lead? Other developed nations all have some form of universal healthcare, so successful advertising of prescription medications would lead to higher but unnecessary costs. In the United States, these increased costs are shifted to the public, and create huge profits for Big Pharma. Those who ask their doctor about a specific drug are more likely to have it prescribed than if they simply presented with symptoms for which that drug might be beneficial(9). Advertising works resulting in widespread unnecessary prescribing.

In our profit-oriented healthcare system, doctors, hospitals clinics, and other healthcare providers promote their services in attention-getting ways. One clinic in Seattle has bus billboards displaying the clinic logo alongside the statement, "When the going gets tough," and in the corner ... "urology." Another uses the catchphrase, "When the shoe no longer fits," with "podiatry" in the corner. I drove behind a van carrying medical imaging equipment. On the back was written, "Detect More Cancers. Save More Lives. It's that simple." Although we do a lot of screening for cancers, other countries save more lives, as demonstrated by their considerably lower overall death rates. Ask yourself, who does all this advertising benefit? Does the advertising make us healthier, or the advertiser richer?

The media shape our perceptions of health, but the healthcare industry doesn't always benefit from that coverage. Media reports of hospitals being overwhelmed with COVID-19 patients and surges in recent variants have led to a marked decline in people seeking medical care in the United States. These drops have resulted in considerable loss of revenue for many healthcare facilities. In response, the medical care industrial complex has stepped up their advertising telling people not to delay such care. Healthcare marketing campaigns stress getting back on the schedule for elective procedures now that restrictions for physical distancing have been relaxed. In a profit-driven healthcare system, marketing campaigns will inevitably shape our perceptions of our healthcare needs and treatment. Yet marketing is just one of many ways that the healthcare industry shapes our health.

Profit-Care or Healthcare?

There is tremendous waste in providing unnecessary medical services to patients. A 2013 Institute of Medicine (IOM) study found over 700 billion dollars in overused and unnecessary healthcare spending in 2009 alone(10). A 2014 survey of physicians validated these findings, revealing that unnecessary tests and over-treatment were commonly a result of the fear of malpractice claims. Almost three quarters of surveyed doctors believed that physicians were more likely to perform unnecessary procedures when they gained financially from them. The survey results indicate roughly a third of tests, procedures, and prescribed medicines were believed to be unnecessary. One emerging way of curbing some of this excess is through virtual care.

In the not too distant past, a doctor talking to a patient on the phone did not represent a medical encounter and could not be billed for, so the practice was discouraged. Instead, you had to make a physical appointment. But in many cases, a patient's health concern can be adequately addressed through video conferencing, such as discussing her sleeplessness, or his flare-up of arthritis. And it can be difficult for some patients to get to a healthcare facility. They may live far away from the facility or lack transportation to get there. Arranging childcare to make the visit possible can be difficult for many. Just taking the time off work for the added travel time can pose a burden for many patients. And with a physical visit, there is likely a greater opportunity to charge more for unneeded physical exams, tests, and procedures and such so costs go up. Finally, the virtual encounter with their doctor, nurse practitioner, or physician's assistant that they have already established a relationship with, can be sufficient and maintains trust in the caring connection, which telemedicine can provide. As we've seen during the pandemic, virtual care can and does work for many, and it is likely here to stay.

Despite the rise in virtual visits, patients still want to go to the doctor. Most Americans believe that more medical care is better, that newer is better, and that you get what you pay for. There seems to be no upper limit to the amount of healthcare people will consume if they can pay for it themselves or have it paid for by insurance.

From a medical standpoint, if you think you are healthy you haven't had enough tests yet! A normal lab value is determined by examining large numbers of people with a given test. Then the middle 95% are deemed normal, and those outside the limits are abnormal. By doing enough investigations, one can always come up with an abnormal lab value or a questionable finding on a scan or test despite there being nothing wrong. This finding leads to further investigations, often done to ensure care has been comprehensive enough to avoid litigation. Besides increasing costs, this process can cause considerable anxiety for patients and can even result in unnecessary deaths.

"Don't just stand there, do something," tends be the way medical care functions. My mantra was, "Don't just do something, stand there—unless there is substantial evidence that doing something is better than not doing it." Common unnecessary procedures include X-rays, CT or MRI scans, or ultrasounds where there is little chance of finding a broken bone and for garden variety back pain, and the prescription of potentially toxic drugs for psychiatric conditions when talk therapy would likely work better, among many others. But too often, a patient didn't want to leave unless they'd felt I'd "done something." In those cases, if I wanted to discharge a patient from the emergency department, an easy way was to give him or her a pharmaceutical prescription.

It's understandable that patients want something done, even when doing nothing resolves ninety percent of all health problems. Much of this perception comes from the trend in evidence-based medicine, which promotes the idea that tests and procedures help.

Evidence-based medicine advances the idea that care should be guided by the results of many studies—especially clinical trials—on what is effective and what is not. However, such studies supplant experience gained in clinical practice which is not accounted for by specific research. Many low-quality studies support evidence-based medicine but are often funded by those who stand to gain economically from the specific treatment that comes out best, such as the maker of the pharmaceutical being studied.

Gauging trends in treatment for COVID-19 is a good example of developing protocols, testing them and coming up with guidelines for evidence-based care. Those with a serious COVID illness typically present with difficulties transporting oxygen from the lungs to the rest of the body. Without oxygen cells and organs die and soon we follow. There are many options for ventilatory support to improve oxygen delivery to the body, but they require good judgment on when to use them. Moreover, a variety of drugs were thought to be effective in stabilizing patients but were later found to not be that useful. We hope drugs will be developed to treat COVID-19. Nonetheless, any doctor can use any legally approved drug for any purpose deemed appropriate. From my perspective, one must rely on a doctor's clinical judgment. This is a difficult path for a COVID-19 patient and their family to navigate, a choice made even more difficult by media reports promoting a variety of unusual treatments for COVID. Also most insurance companies will not cover the cost of a drug or treatment that is used for an unapproved purpose.

As these examples show, the care you receive when you go to the doctor or hospital is shaped by an industry aimed at making profit—and by your own perceptions, themselves shaped by media messaging and advertising. But what happens to your health when you do get treated?

Effects of Medical Treatments

Medical care can diagnose illness and injury, but a lack of medical care is not the cause of illness or injury. Medicine is more an art than a science. State-of-the-art care changes over time. When I was in medical school in 1972, a professor of medicine began his lecture by informing us that, "In ten years' time you will discover that half of what I am telling you is wrong. I just don't know which half."

We didn't give aspirin to someone having a heart attack until after 1980, but it's now routinely administered even before the victim gets to the hospital. Until the 2000s, post-menopausal women were given estrogen to replace the hormones they no longer produced, with one study finding slight gains in life expectancy from the use of that therapy. We now know this practice to be harmful.

I received standard of care radiation for facial acne as a teenager in the 1950s. It cleared up my acne and I was thrilled, but that treatment later led to lymph gland cancer, which still plagues me today. Radiation was used to treat many other conditions in the past: asthma, sinus conditions, enlarged tonsils, and heavy menses. These treatments have been abandoned because we now know the harm they cause. Which of our current state-of-the-art practices will be seen as harmful in a few decades?

Consider medical care comparisons across nations for conditions that should be responsive to care. Although for many conditions medical care has little to offer, there are many others for which it is beneficial: bacterial infections, diabetes, heart attacks, HIV/AIDS, hypertension, maternal bleeding during delivery, and leukemia in young people. The United States performs badly even for those problems: repeated studies show we have considerably higher mortality for treatable conditions than other rich nations. Although deaths from these situations are decreasing overall, the improvements are unfortunately shameful in the United States. Comparing avoidable deaths and 10-year mortality reduction (2009–19) among rich countries, the Commonwealth Fund shows the United States as the worst(11). Why are the deficiencies of medical care are not stressed? Because they would compete with the victories of healthcare.

We doctors pride ourselves on "saving lives." I recall attending my first emergency code as a medical student at Stanford. Someone's heart stopped beating and a physician-in-training administered a defibrillating shock that restarted the heart. After the chief resident arrived, he asked who shocked the patient. A hand motioned, and he said solemnly, "You saved a life." Saving lives, seeded in my mind as a child, is the metaphor of medical care. But is it true? In too many cases, it isn't medical care that does the saving.

As a medical intern one evening in 1973, I looked at an issue of the *Journal of Infectious Diseases*, containing an article by Edward Kass, a renowned infectious diseases doctor at Harvard(12). In that article "Infectious Diseases and Social Change," Kass presented data on deaths from various infectious diseases since the 1850s in England and Wales, where reliable records had been kept. He noted that poorer people were consistently more likely to succumb to infections. Considering tuberculosis, diphtheria, scarlet fever, measles, and whooping cough, he then presented data demonstrating that deaths from these problems dropped profoundly even before the advent of antibiotics or immunizations. Kass argued that this decline in deaths resulted from improvements in socioeconomic circumstances and standards of living, not medical care. He called it "the most important happening in the history of the health of man." It took a few decades for the concepts I read that day to sink in, but Kass' article prompted me to start asking important questions. One of those questions was, how can we distinguish medical care's benefit from threat?

Medical Harm

Consider giving two groups of people different levels of medical care, with one group receiving as much free care as they want and the other having to co-pay part of the cost. In the Rand Health Insurance Study, over 4,000 adults were randomly assigned to one of these two groups(13). Those who had to pay part of the cost of their care used a third fewer services and had a third fewer hospitalizations than those who had free care. The result? Essentially no differences in mortality rates.

A more extreme version of this approach considers what happens to death rates when doctors go on strike(14). Mortality declines when doctors don't go to work. One study of people receiving less treatment because of a doctor's strike was done for the month-long anesthesiologists' 1976 strike in Los Angeles County. County coroner death rates fell during the strike. Deaths then increased afterwards as elective surgeries had been postponed.

This unexpected finding, that less care is not really less health, has been confirmed again and again, but the reasons behind it are not clear. One possible explanation is that whenever medical care itself has been considered as a possible cause of death, it is always one of the leading factors.

The first major study on medical harm was published in 1991(15). Investigators from Harvard Medical School reviewed a sample of charts from New York hospitals for 1984, documenting "adverse events" that resulted from the care provided. Common problems were reactions to prescribed drugs and surgical wound infections. There were complications from technical procedures, such as leaving an instrument in the body during surgery, or a device not functioning correctly. Adverse events were found to be common, with a substantial proportion ending in death.

Since then, many studies in different countries by different investigators have found medical harm to be common. A key finding: being admitted to a hospital can result in a substantial risk of dying from treatment alone, and the sicker you are and the longer you stay, the greater the risk.

People die in their quest for medical care. The numbers of these deaths vary. In the 2015 issue of *Best Hospitals* from *U.S. News and World Report*, an article on patient safety disclosed that "one analysis put the number of preventable deaths alone each year at 440,0000." In 2016, a study by surgeons at Johns Hopkins University presented medical error as the third leading cause of death in America(16). *The New York Times* reported in 1998 that over 100,000 people die each year from adverse drug reactions (17).

Media attention to the roughly 500,000 treatment-related deaths a year in the United States is scant. Contrast this disinterest with police killings here which now number close to a thousand a year. These avoidable deaths get substantial media coverage. While such coverage is justified, another carnage produces five hundred times more deaths and deserves much more media attention than it receives.

Fortunately, attention is rising. Consider the 2020 title, *When We Do Harm: A Doctor Confronts Medical Error* by a physician at New York's Bellevue Hospital(18). The legal perspective from law professors is presented in, *Closing Death's Door: Legal Innovations to End the Epidemic of Healthcare Harm*(19). Even though I have been harmed by medical care myself, and I have harmed others by providing such care, I shudder to confront this idea. We can only speculate on what impact COVID-19 has on medical harm. Since fewer people received medical care in 2020 in America, perhaps there has been a net benefit. We can hope that only the really sick got treatment and that treatment was for conditions that would benefit by medical care. The research to answer this question has yet to emerge.

Why Are the Effects of Medical Care So Limited?

In addition to the trends in "evidence-based medicine" has come the recent focus on "patient-centered medicine" which claims to rise above disease models and care for whole persons. Body parts are what medical care mostly treats. Take a typical homeless man who I might see in the emergency department, coming in with symptoms of persistent weakness and dizziness for the past six months. Because he'd been admitted through the emergency department—a common source of medical care for people without insurance—he must be screened to make sure there isn't a condition requiring urgent hospital admission. This process takes hours and costs thousands of dollars. Usually there is nothing that justifies a hospital stay, so I have no choice but to send him back out on the street to deal with his problems himself. If healthcare was structured to better address the whole person who, in this case, suffers from extreme social and economic challenges, he could at least be offered a meal and a shower—or, even better, an overnight stay and support in finding housing or a job. But those items are not in the hospital formulary that lists which treatments or drugs can be prescribed.

So medical care essentially treats organs and their component cells, rather than the whole person in need of care. Instead of the help he really needs, the homeless man can be prescribed a medicine to act on vestibular cells to help his dizziness, and perhaps an antidepressant acting on neuron cells in the brain to stabilize his general malaise. But those interventions are treating his cells rather than the whole person. And he is unlikely to have money to pay for those drugs.

If the same homeless person comes in with a heart attack, he will be sent to the cardiac catheterization lab where roto-rooter plumbing can be done to open the blockage in the coronary artery. Unlike in the other scenario, he will be admitted to the hospital. But because he is poor, he will most likely experience complications, including re-blockage at some relatively early point in the future as we will see in Chapter 4. We are treating an organ, not the person himself.

This body part perspective is reflected in major national organizations such as the American Heart Association, and others by the American Lung Association and the National Kidney Foundation. Our body parts have their own lobbying groups to garner money and sympathy. Our national government with its National Cancer Institute, the National Eye Institute, the National Heart, Lung and Blood Institute focuses on diseases as does the National Institute of Allergy and Infectious Diseases with its renown director Dr. Anthony Fauci during our COVID-19 era. We are fixated on body parts and their diseases rather than individual humans.

Consider society's health problems as an overflowing sink. Picture a large room with a sink against one wall. Water is pouring out of the faucet and spilling all over the floor. Two workers dressed in white lab coats are hard at work wiping up the water with mops, but they can't keep up with the endless flow of water. What else needs to be done? The faucet must be turned off. Perhaps the drain should be checked for clogging as well. But this is not the moppers' job, so the flood continues unabated. Are healthcare workers supposed to produce health in society, or are we meant to rely on cleanup medicine, just mopping up the ongoing overflow? When I present this image to students, I ask whose job it is to stop the flow. There is no correct answer, because there is no such job description in this country.

Universal Healthcare

Access to healthcare is a basic human right and an investment in society, as well as enhancing social and economic equity. Yet the United States is the only rich nation today that does not allow everyone to obtain needed medical care. Better access to healthcare services should produce better health but the reality may not be so. What do we know about specific health benefits of universal healthcare at the population level? The information is mixed at best.

Few published studies evaluate the overall health and mortality outcomes of providing universal healthcare. One of the few was carried out in Winnipeg, Canada, looking at data from 1986 to 1996 when all residents had full access to care(20). The researchers were interested in determining whether use of healthcare reduced the inequalities in health outcomes between those with more education and those with less. They also looked at income, dividing those who were hospitalized into groups representing equal fifths of the city's income levels. The results were clear: much more healthcare was consumed by those in less educated neighborhoods, including more doctor contacts, hospital stays, surgeries, and pharmaceuticals. Those with the lowest incomes received more medical care than the next lowest, and so on up the ladder. However, despite the heavy use of medical care, mortality followed the same gradient: residents of the least educated and poorest neighborhoods had the highest death rates and the shortest life expectancy.

The researchers concluded:

> .... a universal health care system is definitely the right policy tool for delivering care to those in need, and for this it must be respected and supported. However, investments in health care should never be confused with, or sold as, policies whose primary intent is to improve population health or to reduce inequalities in health. Claims to that effect are misleading at best, dangerous and highly wasteful at worst.

Healthcare has limited benefits in improving health for people at the lowest social and economic levels in a society. The reasons are clear: poorer people tend to be sicker. The sociopolitical structure of a society determines who gets rich and who stays poor, and there is ample evidence that how you rank in those socioeconomic measures matters the most for your health—the focus of the next chapter.

In 1966, the United States introduced Medicare, which provided universal healthcare coverage for those over age 65. Several studies of the impact of this policy reported substantial economic benefits, meaning less out-of-pocket medical expenditures for senior citizens. However, for the first 10 years, no mortality benefit could be ascribed to this new program. The conclusion: Medicare provides access to important services, but may not improve health for the oldest age group(21).

Another policy experiment took place in Massachusetts. Beginning in 2006, the state policy mandated that nearly all residents were required to have private healthcare insurance, managed through a variety of payment mechanisms, including providing it at no cost to those below a specific poverty level. Comparing Massachusetts adults covered under the plan to uninsured residents of other states with similar characteristics, the plan has shown a small but measurable mortality benefit(22). The gains appear greatest for medical conditions most amenable to medical care, as might be expected for people with lower incomes, including those who were uninsured before the policy change. So in this example, having insurance was associated with a modest improvement in death rates. It also demonstrated the common finding of an increased need for care experienced by those lower on the socioeconomic ladder.

Medicaid is the U.S. program funded by federal and state agencies that covers medical expenses, with varying support, for low income people. The so-called Oregon Experiment in 2008 involved Medicaid expansion in which some adults were assigned by lottery to receive medical coverage, comparing the results with others whose healthcare access remained unchanged(23). The program's first 2 years found improvements in self-rated health, a measure that was used because people's opinion of their own health predicts their mortality risk. There were, however, no significant improvements in measurable physical health, such as lowered blood pressure, cholesterol, or glycated hemoglobin (for those with diabetes). In this program, the use of healthcare services increased, as expected, and individual financial strain was reduced. The conclusions here is that increased access to healthcare probably had some health benefits, but immediate changes were not obvious.

The Affordable Care Act has received constant media attention since its passage in 2010. This complex legislation included several elements. It prevented healthcare insurers from refusing coverage to patients with pre-existing conditions or charging them more. It made purchase of insurance mandatory for certain categories of people, requiring most employers to provide coverage or pay a surtax, and provided low- and middle-income Americans subsidies for the purchase of insurance. The plan also included an expansion of Medicaid to more low-income people, optional at the state level. Toward the end of 2021, some 12 states have chosen to not expand Medicaid, despite the federal government picking up the costs. States that used the Medicaid expansion option have found modest improvements in self-rated health, and more people report accessing medical care than previously. Some benefits seen were that men were more likely to be tested for HIV and more likely to schedule dental visits. The ACA has found that healthcare access increased among poorer people following coverage, so the difference in accessibility between richer and poorer decreased(24). Given the scale of medical costs for the uninsured in this country, the ACA has been cost-saving for many.

A 2017 study by Woolhandler and Himmelstein reviewed research on the link between having healthcare insurance and lower mortality, mostly focusing on the United States(25). Their paper aimed to explain and strengthen the argument made in an earlier IOM report that found that healthcare insurance saves 18,000 lives in the United States (which some researchers had described as over-estimates). Their results confirmed that the chance of dying for the uninsured was significantly greater than for those who had healthcare insurance.

But was it access to healthcare that made the difference? The uninsured were more likely to have lower incomes so it may be that their living conditions made them even more vulnerable to illness and death than those better off. Because of the difficulty of studying the effects of insurance on subpopulations, such as children and the poor, this question has not been definitively answered.

Thus far, a few studies have suggested that universal healthcare coverage may have mortality benefits. But "suggest" and "may have" are important caveats. If medical care does make an important difference in decreasing mortality, it is certainly difficult to demonstrate that effect consistently. In fact, since the inception of the ACA in 2010, death rates in the United States for most groups have risen.

It may be that high rates of medical harm are responsible for the difficulty in demonstrating health benefits, as well as medical care's focus on treating cells and organs rather than on the individual. The benefits of care are probably greatest for children and for poorer people. I agree with the critical need for a single-payer universal healthcare program for everyone in the United States. However, if it were to be put into place tomorrow, that program wouldn't do much to change the key issues addressed in this book. Despite all the medical care we provide, our poor health status continues to be inferior to that of the other rich nations—and before COVID-19 was actually getting worse, that is mortality was increasing. The pandemic has exacerbated the mortality crisis.

I often present the limitations of medical care in improving health to various student groups. One recent study estimated the contribution of healthcare to U.S. longevity on the order of 10%, which is consistent with other such efforts(26). Another review considered the extremely limited benefits of statin use in postponing death(27). People find this difficult to comprehend but these are the facts.

We should have universal healthcare as a human right in the United States. But healthcare is not the major force producing health in a population. This concept is one of the most difficult for people in the United States to grasp. So far, we have been considering healthcare as a monolith and asking what good it does. What if we look now at the components of that pillar to see if one particular portion is beneficial for health? Is there a subset of medical care that can be shown to improve health? Let us consider one particular column of our healthcare system, primary healthcare.

Primary Healthcare

Primary healthcare is the provision of integrated, accessible healthcare services by clinicians who are accountable for addressing a large majority of personal healthcare needs, developing a sustained partnership with patients and with families. This means having a doctor, or other healthcare worker, to whom we turn to get healthcare for most of our illness and preventive healthcare needs. This person is there for us over long periods and works near us. Such a person may have been present when we were born, we turned to them when we were children, and they would be available later in life as we got sick. A family practice doctor or physician's assistant or family nurse practitioner provides this care, although internists and pediatricians also do so.

In the United States, most believe that better care is provided by specialists—nephrologists, cardiologists, cardiac surgeons, or endocrinologists—rather than a family doctor or generalist who practices primary healthcare. We have many more specialists than primary care doctors in this country. Most medical students say they want to pursue esoteric specialties. Why? Partly because they aim to be highly compensated without having to work the long and irregular hours that primary care requires. They are also inspired when they learn that a specific area of medical care will allow them to perform a few procedures very well. Being a generalist who knows enough about a range of health problems is not considered as intellectually satisfying as gaining expertise in a narrower field. Even the terms, generalist, or GP, which can refer to those doing General Practice in the United Kingdom, and is a common term elsewhere, carry disdain in this country. "What? You didn't go to an infectious disease specialist with your cold?" A specialist is seen as preferable.

Studies looking at primary care physicians among U.S. counties from 2005 to 2015 found that where the density of such doctors increased, life expectancy increased as well. But where their proportion to population decreased, life expectancy declined(28). This confirms the importance of primary healthcare to improve health in the United States. Since our health has been declining in the country overall, a part of the reason is that fewer doctors provide primary care services here. The countries with the healthiest populations have three times the proportion of general practitioners or primary care doctors as we do(7). Although the totality of medical care can't adequately counter the corrosive health effects of social and economic hardships, access to quality primary care offers an important way of influencing mortality outcomes.

Public Health

What is public health, and what is its role in producing health? In the United States, the phrase "public health" is generally considered to be something that benefits everybody. Others say public health is public toilets! On their website, the American Public Health Association claims public health "promotes and protects the health of people and the communities where they live, learn, work, and play."

The science of public health has evolved since the 18th century, when it focused on isolating the ill and quarantining those exposed to diseases to prevent transmission of infection. In the 19th century, the focus was on sanitation, especially separating fecal contamination from food and water. Living conditions improved tremendously as a result. With the understanding of infectious disease transmission in the early part of the 20th century, the focus shifted to immunizations and infection control. Later efforts centered on tobacco regulation and decreasing risk factors for chronic diseases such as heart disease and diabetes by promoting diet change and exercise. Efforts were also made to improve workplace conditions and motor vehicle safety. Such programs had definite health benefits that we take for granted today.

What directions should U.S. public health take today to continue health improvements? The IOM's 1988 report, *The Future of Public Health*, distilled its efforts into three pillars: assessment, policy development, and assurance(29). Translated, this means figuring out what the issues or problems are (assessment), doing something about them (policy development), and finally making sure the expected good outcomes occur (assurance). Has this approach been successful?

Assessment in the report asks for critical data collection at the local level: cities, counties, and states. These data include vital statistics such as births and deaths, a state responsibility. Other needed data are disease and health-related behavior surveys. While the Center for Disease Control and Prevention (CDC) collects these data and makes them available to the public, they present almost no comparisons to assessments in other countries. If we search the CDC website for life expectancy, we can see trends in the country and stratification by race/ethnicity subgroups. For maternal mortality, the CDC says that maternal mortality is increasing for 2019 over 2018 and Blacks are most impacted at almost four times the rate for Latinx. Infant mortality (IMR) is stated as being a good indicator of the overall health of a population and the website points out the IMR has dropped from 2017 to 2018, supposedly a good sign.

How does the CDC report American international rankings in recent years. The CDC's *Health USA* report from 1960 to 2016 presented IMR rate and life expectancy data for OECD nations. The United States ranked 11th in 1960 but 24th in 2013! For subsequent reports, those rankings are no longer present although available on the CDC website for 2017 but not 2018. Why have they been omitted? The latest report for 2019 didn't appear until the spring of 2021 when the CDC leadership had changed with the new federal administration. Yet still, there were no international comparisons.

In the IOM's 2003 follow-up report, *The Future of the Public's Health in the 21st Century*, the first chapter launched into "Achievement and Disappointment. "For years, the life expectancies of both men and women in the United States have lagged behind those of their counterparts in most other industrialized nations." Although they recognized the relative decline of the U.S. health compared to other nations, nowhere in their 34 policy recommendations for the future, did they suggest monitoring those trends(30).

There has been no comprehensive follow-up report along these lines looking at organized or institutionalized public health in the United States. Public health services have been drastically defunded throughout the United States. This reduction in services is in part responsible for our dismal COVID-19 mortality.

As our health status has continued to deteriorate in comparison to other countries, rarely do health or mainstream media publications acknowledge that astounding reality even in the COVIDian era. Public health has failed this nation, with its silence on our relatively low health status compared to what we know is possible. The U.S. life expectancy and mortality rates have taken a turn for the worse. Public health is silent on what will be required to reduce this unprecedented, alarming trend.

When you ask people a general question of what can be done to improve health in this country responses tend to be, "focus on prevention." But what is "prevention?" There are three common terms, primary, second, and tertiary prevention. Primary prevention halts the acquisition of a disease such as an immunization against polio. This makes us think in terms of diseases rather than of health. Secondary prevention refers to halting or slowing the progression of a disease once you have acquired it, such as catching breast cancer, or COVID-19 early. Then there is tertiary prevention to halt or reverse or delay disease progression, such as taking statins after a heart attack or dexamethasone for advanced COVID-19. Some have called for quaternary prevention, namely, limiting the harms of healthcare. Another concept is primordial prevention—preventing the emergence of predisposing social and environmental conditions that lead to disease or worse health(31). We have failed for all categories of prevention.

Conclusion

Spending on healthcare has not produced health. Our focus in this book is on primordial prevention, namely, situating health as the cornerstone we must lay. Yes, we need to provide medical care and engage in the other forms of prevention by various means. But that is only the beginning.

In the next chapter, we begin the journey of understanding why our health lags behind that of so many other nations. Does economic inequality kill or is it what makes America so great?

Questions to Consider and Discuss

1. With the medical industrial complex such a powerful entity, not only in America but around the world, how can we take on an alternative model to the biomedical one that impacts our lives in ways that are not healthy?
2. What can be done about the high rate of deaths from medical harm, both in the United States and elsewhere?

Notes

1. Latin for "first do no harm" attributed to Hippocrates. It is the oath many American medical students take when they become doctors.
2. Federal Emergency Management Agency provides funeral and rent assistance and vaccine support while Coronavirus Aid Relief and Economic Security Act (CARES act) passed in 2020 was a $2.2 trillion economic stimulus bill that produced questionable overall benefits for the most vulnerable.

References

1. Kliff S, Katz J. Hospitals and Insurers Didn't Want You to See These Prices. Here's Why.: New York Times; 2021 [cited 2021 August 22]. Available from: https://www.nytimes.com/interactive/2021/08/22/upshot/hospital-prices.html.
2. Dickman S, Mirza R, Kandi M, Incze MA, Dodbiba L, Yameen R, et al. Mortality at For-Profit Versus Not-For-Profit Hemodialysis Centers: A Systematic Review and Meta-Analysis. International Journal of Health Services. 2021;51(3):371–8.
3. Foley RN, Hakim RM. Why Is the Mortality of Dialysis Patients in the United States Much Higher than the Rest of the World? Journal of the American Society of Nephrology. 2009;20(7):1432–5.
4. Himmelstein DU, Campbell T, Woolhandler S. Health Care Administrative Costs in the United States and Canada, 2017. Annals of Internal Medicine. 2020;172(2):134–42.
5. Bunker JP, Frazier HS, Mosteller F. Improving Health: Measuring Effects of Health Care. Milbank Quarterly. 1994;72(2):225–58.
6. Cutler D, Miller G. The Role of Public Health Improvements in Health Advances: The Twentieth-Century United States. Demography. 2005;42(1):1–22.
7. OECD. Health at a Glance 2017: OECD Indicators. Paris: Organisation for Economic, Co-operation and Development; 2017.

8. Briggs CL, Hallin DC. Making Health Public: How News Coverage Is Remaking media, Medicine, and Contemporary Life. Hallin DC, editor. New York, NY: Routledge; 2016.

9. Kravitz RL, Epstein RM, Feldman MD, Franz CE, Azari R, Wilkes MS, et al. Influence of Patients' Requests for Direct-to-Consumer Advertised Antidepressants: A Randomized Controlled Trial. JAMA. 2005;293(16):1995–2002.

10. Institute of Medicine. Best Care at Lower Cost: the Path to Continuously Learning Health Care in America: National Academies Press; 2013.

11. Schneider EC, Shah A, Doty MM, Tikkanen R, Fields K, Williams II RD. Mirror, Mirror 2021: Reflecting Poorly Health Care in the US Compared to Other High-Income Countries. New York, NY: The Commonwealth Fund; 2021 August 4.

12. Kass EH. Infectious Diseases and Social Change. Journal of Infectious Diseases. 1971; 123(1):110–4.

13. Ware J, Brook R, Rogers W, Keeler EB, Davies AR, Sherbourne CD, et al. Health Outcomes for Adults in Prepaid and Fee-for-Service Care: Results from the Health Insurance Experiment. Santa Monica, CA: Rand Corporation; 1987.

14. Cunningham SA, Mitchell K, Narayan KM, Yusuf S. Doctors' Strikes and Mortality: a Review. Social Science & Medicine. 2008;67(11):1784–8.

15. Brennan TA, Leape LL, Laird NM, Hebert L, Localio AR, Lawthers AG, et al. Incidence of Adverse Events and Negligence in Hospitalized Patients. Results of the Harvard Medical Practice Study I. New England Journal of Medicine. 1991;324(6):370–6.

16. Makary MA, Daniel M. Medical Error—the Third Leading Cause of Death in the US. BMJ. 2016;353:i2139.

17. Lazarou J, Pomeranz BH, Corey PN. Incidence of Adverse Drug Reactions in Hospitalized Patients: a Meta-Analysis of Prospective Studies. JAMA. 1998;279(15):1200–5.

18. Ofri D. When We Do Harm: a Doctor Confronts Medical Error. Boston: Beacon; 2020.

19. Saks MJ, Landsman S. Closing Death's Door: Legal Innovations to End the Epidemic of Healthcare Harm. Landsman S, editor. New York, NY: Oxford University Press; 2021.

20. Roos NP, Brownell M, Menec V. Universal Medical Care and Health Inequalities: Right Objectives, Insufficient Tools. In: Heymann J, Hertzman C, Barer ML, Evans RG, editors. Healthier Societies: From Analysis to Action. New York, NY: Oxford University Press; 2006. pp. 107–31.

21. Finkelstein A, McKnight R. What Did Medicare Do? The Initial Impact of Medicare on Mortality and Out of Pocket Medical Spending. Journal of Public Economics. 2008;92(7):1644–68.

22. Sommers BD, Long SK, Baicker K. Changes in Mortality After Massachusetts Health Care Reform: A Quasi-experimental Study. Annals of Internal Medicine. 2014;160(9): 585–93.

23. Baicker K, Taubman SL, Allen HL, Bernstein M, Gruber JH, Newhouse JP, et al. The Oregon Experiment—Effects of Medicaid on Clinical Outcomes. New England Journal of Medicine. 2013;368(18):1713–22.

24. Soni A, Wherry LR, Simon KI. How Have ACA Insurance Expansions Affected Health Outcomes? Findings From The Literature. Health Affairs. 2020;39(3):371–8.

25. Woolhandler S, Himmelstein DU. The Relationship of Health Insurance and Mortality: Is Lack of Insurance Deadly? Annals of Internal Medicine. 2017;167(6):424–31.

26. Kaplan, RM, Milstein, A. Contributions of Health Care to Longevity: A Review of 4 Estimation Methods. Annals of Family Medicine. 2019;17:267–72.

27. Hansen, MR, Hróbjartsson, A, Pottegård, A, Damkier, P, Larsen, KS, Madsen, KG, dePont Christensen, R, Kristensen, MEL, Christensen, PM, Hallas, J. Postponement of Death by Statin Use: A Systematic Review and Meta-Analysis of Randomized Clinical Trials. Journal of General Internal Medicine. 2019;34(8):1607–14.

28. Basu S, Berkowitz SA, Phillips RL, Bitton A, Landon BE, Phillips RS. Association of Primary Care Physician Supply with Population Mortality in the United States, 2005–2015. JAMA Internal Medicine. 2019;179(4):506–14.

29. Institute of Medicine. The Future of Public Health. Washington, D.C.: National Academy Press; 1988.

30. Institute of Medicine. The Future of the Public's Health in the 21st Century. Washington, D.C.: National Academy Press; 2003.

31. Starfield B, Hyde J, Gervas J, Heath I. The Concept of Prevention: A Good Idea Gone Astray? Journal of Epidemiology and Community Health. 2008;62(7):580–3.

Chapter 3

Inequality Kills

> I believe that virtually all the problems in the world come from inequality of one kind or another.
>
> *Amartya Sen (Nobel-prize winning economist)*

In Chapter 1, I used the term "Health Olympics." My conclusion: if health were an Olympic event, and countries were ranked by a range of mortality measures, the United States would be behind around 50 other nations, depending on the indicator used. The evidence is overwhelming that we cannot boast of being healthy if the standard is comparing ourselves to those living in other industrialized and low-middle income countries. Since 2015, and before COVID, our health had been declining absolutely, with a decreasing length of life and increasing mortality. COVID-19 has further increased our health gap with other nations. These killer facts should be disturbing to all Americans.

This chapter will show how such economic inequality undermines our health through the social stress that impacts our lives and our well-being. Economic inequality also creates a society in which richer folk influence the political process to pollute the situation for the rest of us. The American COVID-19 predicament has strongly reinforced these uneven impacts, and without changing course, the consequences will only worsen.

Upstream at the Source

An allegory that has been told for many decades distinguishes upstream from downstream factors.

Imagine, if you will, three people standing alongside a river on a brisk afternoon. They suddenly hear a cry for help from someone caught in the river's fast-moving current.

Our three bystanders react in different ways.

The first bystander becomes angry at the unfortunate person's irresponsibility.

"Don't you know how to swim?" this bystander shouts. "You never should have jumped in!"

DOI: 10.4324/9781003315889-4

The second bystander wants to be more helpful. She waves to our desperate victim and displays a discount coupon for swimming lessons. "Quick, grab this," she pleas, "With this you'll be able to afford the lessons!"

Finally, our third bystander—a rescue worker—jumps in the water and pulls the flailing floater out of the water. Paramedics soon make it to the scene. They administer CPR and transport the victim to the hospital.

That rescue, unfortunately, doesn't end the crisis. The next day sees more thrashing people floating down the river and more still the day after. Researchers take notice. They start tabulating how many people are floating by. They survey the survivors, compare their educational levels and race, and construct elaborate personal risk-taking profiles. But this research doesn't stem the tide of flailing floaters. Pulling them out of the water is rapidly becoming an expensive proposition. Just extracting victims from the river, people soon realize, is never going to eliminate the problem. Too many keep falling in!

What's causing all the tragic river traffic? No one really knows. A few public health workers decide to head upstream to find out. They soon spot billboards with glamorous and fetching pictures marketing the river's many recreational opportunities. One public health worker concludes that legislation is needed to require all riverside billboards to carry notices warning people about the rapid river currents.

But another contends that warning notices won't be enough and recommends a ban on all billboards as a means of protecting those most vulnerable to the marketing messages.

Executives of the river billboard association quickly erupt in predictable fury. They can't believe what they're hearing. "We demand freedom of speech!" they cry. "Let's not allow people who can't swim to ruin the fun for everybody else!"

"Amen," chimes in the local newspaper editor. "We don't need new government regulations." The responsibility for river safety lies with families, not the government.

This back-and-forth debate frustrates still other public health workers on the original fact-finding mission up the river. They opt to continue even farther up the river and discover that the riverbanks where people walk have eroded into steep and slippery, uneven slopes. No one walking these banks can gain a stable foothold.

At the steepest points of the riverbank, desperate people are even pushing others into the water to secure their own safety. In less steep sections, the public health workers see less chaos. People in these somewhat safer spots seem more secure. Some of them are even helping those around them negotiate the hazardous terrain.

The diligent public health workers soon see a solution. They proceed to build a retaining wall that enables everybody to walk safely along the river. They also excavate some of the steepest parts of the slope to make it safer for all. In short order, no one's flailing in the water anymore.

Does anything in this story sound familiar? Has our path become more secure over time? Have we become safer? One answer lies in reflecting on how COVID-19 has impacted our path to personal and public health.

Economic Inequality as the Driver of Population Health

What's the steep slope at the upstream source that is wreaking havoc with health in the United States? Consider it the gradient between the richest and poorest people in the United States How steep is it in other nations?

A person who knows only one country knows no country. To understand a phenomenon requires comparing it to others. Living in another country for a considerable time and interacting with the people and their culture in some meaningful way can produce useful insights into our own people and culture. My time spent in Nepal, about ten years in total, has been one of my most formative experiences. Nepal is renowned for its geographical slopes but when it comes to social gradients, the steepness of the slope between its richest and poorest is much less than that of Mount Everest. In the United States, however, our incline is stratospheric! How did I come to recognize how important the difference between these two countries is in terms of our health?

By 1991, I knew that quite a few countries had lower mortality and longer life spans than the United States. In 1992, hoping to explain the persistent health decline in the United States relative to other rich nations, I studied at the Johns Hopkins School of Hygiene and Public Health. I was surprised to find no faculty there who were comparing U.S. health with that of other nations. Asking professors why produced responses that there was no funding for that kind of research. I rediscovered there the truism that money talks, at least when the conversation is about what questions are asked and what answers sought. That education also helped me to recognize the major roles social and political forces have in producing health.

In 1992, a publication appeared in the *British Medical Journal* written by Richard Wilkinson, featuring a simple graph of life expectancy in 1981 among nine rich nations, along with the percentage of income received by the poorest 70% of families for each country(1). It showed how greater inequality in a country was associated with lower life expectancy, with only a weak link between national incomes and mortality rates. Richer countries were not necessarily healthier than less rich ones, at least among developed nations. Increases in income inequality over time were linked to higher death rates. But were the results valid?

Depending on a single study as definitive evidence is a shaky way to stake a claim. Knowledge progresses by conjectures, critical commentary, discussions, and either general acceptance or rejection. Yet five previous studies, beginning in 1979, demonstrate similar findings. In 1996, two studies from University of California and Harvard reported the same finding within the United States: more unequal states had higher mortality(2, 3). Later research showed the same result for large U.S. cities(4).

That same year, a landmark book, *Unhealthy Societies: The Afflictions of Inequality,* by Wilkinson appeared expounding these concepts(5). My own heavily annotated copy reflects the importance of this book as a huge step toward recognizing the effect of the social environment on health, while more recently, COVID-19 has highlighted the critical role social policies play in human survival. Similar studies link U.S. state and county death rates associated with COVID-19 with income inequality. The first paper found that more unequal states had higher COVID-19 death rates(6). In June 2021, a study showing U.S. counties with higher income inequality had higher rates of COVID cases and deaths(7). While the British media, with a July 2021 article in *The Economist,* pinpointed these studies, the U.S. media has mostly been silent. One subsequent study of 84 countries found more COVID-19 deaths associated with increasing economic inequality. Even a small rise in inequality gives rise to a substantial increase in COVID-19 deaths(8). Income inequality has soared with the pandemic providing other incriminating evidence that it kills. Still, correlation doesn't imply causation. How do we know that something causes something else?

The U.S. Surgeon General's 1964 report, *Smoking and Health,* outlined the criteria for inferring that something, in this case, cigarettes, caused something, in this case, worse health(9). The criteria were straightforward. First, there had to be many studies demonstrating the relationship, by different investigators, on different populations, over different time periods. Then the chicken and egg problem had to be addressed: did people start smoking and then their health worsened, or was it the other way around—their health got worse so they started smoking? Third, were there other better explanations for the association? Finally, was there some type of biological plausibility, namely, a mechanism through which smoking produced worse health?

By 1964, we had conclusive evidence that all these conditions were met for tobacco as damaging to health. Today, using the same criteria, we can state that inequality in a population causes worse health.

Kate Pickett and Richard Wilkinson pointed out that criteria for a causal relationship are met(10). The strong links of economic inequality to vital aspects of society, including health, are supported by solid research findings. As in the tobacco case, however, widespread acceptance of the inequality-health relationship takes time.

How Does Economic Inequality Affect Health?

Demonstrating the association between more economic inequality and worse health depends on multiple factors. One needs a threshold of income inequality—it must be greater than a certain magnitude before the relationship is observed. For relatively equal nations, the health effects aren't apparent. There may be a lag between increases in income inequality and associated health outcomes. For small geographic groups, a small neighborhood, for example, people tend to live among others like themselves, so it would be unlikely that inequality and health would be associated there. Nevertheless, science shows that inequality is bad for health.

Yet despite overwhelming evidence of our progress in technologies that have transformed our lives, as well as our understanding of biology, disease transmission, and genetics, some people are still suspicious of "science." Perhaps a quarter of adults in the United States have said in surveys that the sun orbits the earth. Ask that question on the internet, and you'll be surprised at what is believed. A third of American Millennials belief the earth is flat according to a 2018 survey report in *Forbes*. A 2005 survey of people's beliefs on evolution in 34 countries published in *Science* found only Turkey had fewer acceptors of the evidence than we have in the United States(11). In today's media climate, misinformation, disinformation, false facts, deep fakes, conspiracy theories, fake news, and many other categories of falsehoods suggest that whatever we believe we can find or purchase our own reality to prove it. In our cyberspace landscape, we can reinforce almost any imaginable thought. Democrats drink baby blood. Hillary Clinton ran a child-sex ring. The COVID vaccine is being secretly slipped into our salad dressing!

Why do many distrust scientific evidence? Because it challenges their beliefs. Recall the epistemology discussion in Chapter 1. Our parents and friends immensely influence what we believe to be true. Today social media is a major influencer, and because we follow accounts of like-minded people, social media serves as echo chambers of our views. If presented with ideas contradicting what is out there that we don't want to believe, we dig in our heels and resist. To say we are not the healthiest country in the world when we know we are the best makes us cover our ears and eyes to not face reality. And income inequality affecting my health? That is just beyond the pale.

However, most of us do consider scientific evidence valuable in helping us understand the world around us. What, then, is the science of economic inequality's relationship with health?

Richard Wilkinson had nudged the inequality-health field into academic prominence after his 1992 paper. Working with Kate Pickett, in 2009 they wrote, *The Spirit Level: Why Greater Equality Makes Societies Stronger*—a popular book linking a variety of health and social problems to income inequality among 23 rich nations, in which they lay out the evidence that inequality kills(12).

The authors created an index of health and social problems that included life expectancy, infant mortality, homicides, mental illness, teenage births, obesity, trust, imprisonment, children's educational performance, and social mobility (Figure 3.1). The index showed a strong relationship between social dysfunction (things we don't want in society) with income inequality among the rich nations. They found that the United States had the most income inequality and the worst outcomes for the index. This seminal book has been translated into many languages and has sold close to a million copies.

Health and social problems are worse in more unequal countries

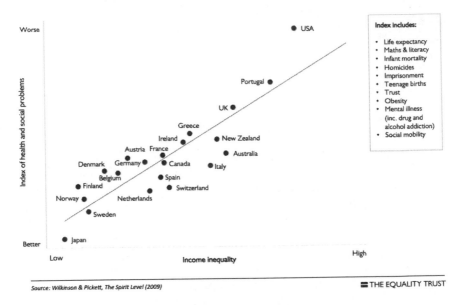

Source: Wilkinson & Pickett, The Spirit Level (2009)   ≡ THE EQUALITY TRUST

Figure 3.1 Health and social problems index related to income inequality(12).

The book's perspective has become more widely known among people outside the United States. Why aren't we listening?

Professors Ichiro Kawachi and S.V. Subramanian of Harvard University address the income inequality health question by presenting three key arguments(13). First there are "diminishing returns" to health with increasing income. Inequality's second impact is through its psychosocial effects, showing that inequality causes stress and frustration leading to worse health. Third, there is a contextual effect of inequality. The rich increasingly control the political process and enjoy policies that benefit them, at the expense of everyone else. Let's explore.

Diminishing Returns

Richer people have better health, as measured by mortality rates, than poorer people. However, adding an additional ten thousand dollars, say, to the income of a very rich person does little or nothing to improve their health, while adding that amount to a poor person's income has substantial health benefits. Such a relationship is observed in nearly all societies.

This trend is clear when looking at death rates for people in the United States by zip code of residence, sorted by the average incomes in each zip code.

Mortality is consistently lower for the richer zip codes than in the poorer ones. A Boston billboard once noted, "Your zip code is more important for your health than your genetic code." In the richest zip codes, mortality doesn't change much at different income levels; the people who live there are all rich. But there are marked differences going from the poorest to the next poorest zip codes and on up. For those groups, a bit of added income can make a big difference in their lives and health. If we take some income from those near the top and give it to those near the bottom, health for those near the top may drop slightly, if at all, but there will be large improvements for those near the bottom. On average the health of the population will be better by redistributing a little from the rich to the poor.

This relationship, diminishing returns to more income, explains only a small part of the American effect of higher income inequality and worse health. Something more powerful is going on, namely, the stress of income comparisons we make. Those with lower incomes experience more.

Psychosocial Effects

Their second link is the psychosocial stress produced by inequality. People may have enough resources to provide for basic needs, which typically include food, water, shelter, and security, but may not have enough to support the more lavish lifestyle that they see others enjoying. With a large income and wealth gap, they recognize what they don't have and compete for higher status. Such an unequal society engenders stress and frustration. We recognize the need to "be nice" to our superiors if we are to keep our job or look good in society.

At the same time, we may put down those below our niche, as exemplified by most Americans' dehumanizing attitude toward the homeless they see with their signs on the streets, asking for help. If we were truly compassionate, we would invite them to our homes or ask to help in other ways, but most turn their heads and walk away. This dehumanization is also observed in social rank ordering in experimental situations. In one study, students were given pictures of others (including homeless, drug addicts, sexualized women, and American Olympic athletes) while in a functional MRI brain scanner to see what kind of activation occurred depending on responses to the pictures regarding pride, envy, pity, or disgust. Pride and envy responses were noted for those considered above the subject's status and pity and disgust at those below(14).

Living in America, we internalize the myth that we are all middle class and have equal opportunities meaning life here is fair. We make comparisons all the time trying to boost our self-esteem. We envy up and scorn down which produces tremendous collateral damage. Envy implies I wish I had what you have, but also that I wish you did not have it. Those we envy have power and are desensitized to the needs of others below them. Scorn means you are unworthy of my attention. We don't help those below us. We are very sensitive to status anxiety.

In a competitive individualistic society, we don't want someone else to get ahead, because it means we have gotten behind. This perception has been reported in many parts of the United States. The competition fostered by inequality is not new. In 1928, the British playwright, George Bernard Shaw, observed(15):

> The woman from the brick box maintains her social position by being offensive to the immense number of people whom she considers her inferiors, reserving her civility for the very few who are clinging to her own little ledge on the social precipice; for inequality of income takes the broad, safe and fertile plain of human society and stands it on edge so that everyone has to cling desperately to her foothold and kick off as many others as she can.

This displaced aggression or "pecking order" has been observed, first in chickens and in other animal societies, such as Macaque monkeys. If a monkey in a group has been the object of aggressive behavior by a higher-ranking individual, the monkey will take it out on one lower in the hierarchy. The one below will in turn take it out on another below him, and so on. The ones at the bottom have no victims for their frustrations. Although being physically put down is not healthy for those at the lowest level, the emotional costs higher up are also important. Your boss gives you a bad evaluation. You won't get angry at the boss because it's risky to do so. Instead, you might go home and shout at your partner. She takes it out on your child. Your child takes it out on a toy, or a friend, or a pet. Today, COVID has produced much more aggressive behavior toward others through such displaced aggression, as domestic abuse skyrockets, violent crime increases, and marriages fall apart. COVID has markedly increased our stress and anxiety. The media, the Center for Disease Control and Prevention (CDC) and various experts abound with advice about how people can cope with this new stress associated with social isolation, economic distress, and the threat of a deadly contagion. Again, those who are in marginalized or down-trodden communities will be less able to manage this challenge because they are more likely to be in low-paying jobs that are more vulnerable to lay-offs, are more likely to live in crowded housing, and be less able to afford assistance with childcare.

Status anxiety, the inevitable outcome of income inequality, is found at all levels of income. The very rich often don't want to talk about their wealth. Rachel Sherman finds that many of the rich don't admit to being more than middle-class, despite having several homes and other trappings of wealth(16). Though objectively very wealthy, they think of those who have even more than they do as "affluent." Michael Milken, the junk bond trader, got on the Forbes Billionaire list some years back. The story goes that when a friend was congratulating him for getting on the list, Milken replied, "But I'm at the bottom!" Pecking order anxieties and frustrations pervade society when there is a large wealth gap.

When I worked as an emergency doctor in a Seattle hospital I occasionally sat in the nearby doctor's lounge between patients. What did my fellow physician colleagues talk about? Not medicine, not family. They would obsess about money. How much others made, and how little they had. As a result, I began counting my money. Once this started, despite having more than I'd ever had before, it seemed I never had enough! I soon recognized the toxic impact of evaluating my resources, and avoided the complaint sessions in the lounge. Then I felt less anxious. And I stopped counting my money. In my current position at a state university, however, I discovered that employee income was publicly available on a website. Seeing for the first time how much greater some incomes were than mine made me feel less worthy. I haven't repeated that inspection. It wasn't a change in income that influenced how I felt about it, it was my perception of that income relative to the income of others. We are, most of us, sensitive to comparing ourselves to others, yet we do so in a multitude of ways, from "keeping up with the Jones's" to evaluating our lives based on how others project their lives on social media.

Among my students, many sense immense stress and competition for what they see as the few opportunities that will come their way after graduation. A large proportion are saddled with huge student debt, while a few, with family support, are spared this concern. Such differences generate considerable status envy. The carefree situation of just a generation or two ago, when even private universities in the United States were relatively inexpensive to attend, is gone.

There is less status anxiety where there are smaller income gaps. One study asked respondents to agree or disagree with the statement, "Some people look down on me because of my job situation or income." Those in more unequal societies were found to have greater status anxiety at any income level than people in places with less inequality(17). There is also less trust in a more unequal society, and we are less likely to cooperate with one another. This results in considerable spending for "security" to guard our resources, yet does increasing our "security" make us feel any better or enhance our well-being?

The social epidemiologist, Sir Michael Marmot, who has done groundbreaking work on the determinants of health, coined the term "status syndrome" to reflect the gradient of poorer health with lower status(18).

To rank status researchers use a ten-step ladder and ask people to place themselves on that ladder(19). The top step represents the highest status and the bottom the lowest. Where subjects place themselves reflects their health status as well. I use this exercise in class, and find my students cluster just above the middle of the ladder. Where would you, the reader, put yourself?

Our perception of ourselves relative to others is central to our well-being. I grew up in a working-class neighborhood where my father repaired shoes, and we lived above the store. While there were some status differences in the community, they were relatively small. I didn't think of myself as poor until I went to Harvard and encountered other students who drove fancy cars, took foreign vacations and acted with a certain arrogance or privilege. Yet I had made friends with high-achieving students. We were all going places upon graduation. As a first-generation university student, my education at elite universities enabled me to perceive my place on the social ladder as rising.

Poverty is a complex concept to be further explored in Chapter 4. Stanford neuroscientist Robert Sapolsky writes, "Given food, shelter, and safety sufficient to sustain health, if everyone is poor, then no one is."(20) Similarly, Karl Marx wrote, "A house may be large or small; as long as the surrounding houses are equally small, it satisfies all social demands for a dwelling. But if a palace rises beside the little house, the little house shrinks into a hut."(21) Our unequal society has us constantly making comparisons and feeling worse for it.

In Nepal I found that the poorer people I met were more inclined to share what little they had than those considerably richer. I lived with people in remote areas who had only the basic material goods they needed but were not aware of what they didn't have. Their moral compass directed them to share. Paul Piff, a Berkeley social psychologist, has carried out a variety of studies on prosocial behavior (sharing, volunteering, helping others) demonstrating lower class people were more trusting, charitable and offered more help. Drivers of high status cars were more likely to cut off other vehicles at intersections and endanger pedestrians at crossings than those in more modest automobiles(22). In countries with less inequality, these behaviors are less likely.

As inequality grows, some boost their status by boasting and other displays of arrogance. More narcissism is seen in more unequal societies. In today's digital era, social media provides endless reinforcement of this trend. Anyone can start a blog to tell the world about their daily lives. Twitter, Facebook, Instagram, and other forms of social media provide a constant forum for showcasing our views, achievements, and even what we ate for breakfast. The result for many at seeing others' displays is feeling worse about their own situations. Good fortune is never enough; others may have it better.

Creating high status body images is an enormous industry in the United States. Relative status within a social group can be displayed by dress and various forms of body adornment such as piercings, tattoos, and hair styles, and by plastic surgery, which is increasingly common among younger and younger American women who desire to look better through surgical enhancement, both above and below the neck. If you can't afford plastic surgery, there are injectables to paralyze our wrinkles, plump our sagging features, and dissolve our double chins. And if you can't afford injectables, there are now many selfie surgery apps to enhance a facial image to look perfect on social media. The desire to look your best begins at increasingly younger ages, with padded bikini tops sold to girls as young as seven. And as the COVID-19 pandemic transforms our face-to-face meetings to Zoom calls, the anxiety of being picture-perfect has led to an increased demand for plastic surgery to enhance our looks on camera(23). How we and others see ourselves has become more important as our social lives shift from those we live alongside of to those we never meet.

This desire for status and respect is not new. Economist Adam Smith in his *The Theory of Moral Sentiments* (1759)(24) wrote:

> To what purpose is all the toil and bustle of this world? What is the end of avarice and ambition, of the pursuit of wealth, of power and pre-eminence? Is it to supply the necessities of nature? The wages of the meanest labourer can supply them... What are the advantages of that great purpose of human life which we call bettering our condition? To be observed, to be attended to, to be taken notice of with sympathy, complacency, and approbation, are all the advantages which we can propose to derive from it. The rich man glories in his riches because he feels that they naturally draw upon him the attention of the world. The poor man on the contrary is ashamed of his poverty. He feels that it places him out of the sight of mankind. To feel that we are taken no notice of necessarily disappoints the most ardent desires of human nature. The poor man goes out and comes in unheeded, and when in the midst of a crowd is in the same obscurity as if shut up in his own hovel. The man of rank and distinction, on the contrary, is observed by all the world. Everybody is eager to look at him. His actions are the objects of the public care. Scarce a word, scarce a gesture that fall from him will be neglected.

Income comparisons reflect status differences. Suppose you are asked to choose between living in a world where your current income is a certain level (say, $50k) and that of others you know is half of yours ($25k), or the opposite scenario where you make $100k but everyone else you know makes $250k. In each case, your income is enough to provide for your needs. Because your purchasing power remains the same, the only difference in your income is what others receive. That is, would you rather have a reasonable income that is double that of your friends/acquaintances, or make a higher amount which is nonetheless considerably less than what others around you make? What do people choose, assuming the purchasing power is the same in each situation? Such an experiment was first carried out in 1995 on public health students at Harvard by Sara Solnick and David Hemenway(25). As they found, and I do repeatedly in my classes, about half the subjects choose the first option, having less but more than everybody else, and the other half are willing to be disadvantaged in comparison with the wealthier. In an unequal society, many want to see themselves as better off than others.

Aggressive or antisocial behavior on airplanes, air rage, reflects our inequality. In such situations, passengers have emotional outbursts, becoming abusive and unruly on the flight(26). A large plane with its differential seating (first class and coach, sometimes a business class) presents physical and situational inequality that affects travelers in each class. On a plane where all passengers enter through the first class cabin, more air rage is seen than if there are no separately classed seats. The angry outbursts will increase in both the first-class and coach sections, but are especially high in first class. There is something stressful to those sitting in first class to have lower class passengers pass by. If entry is in the middle of the plane, as on some jumbo jets, then air rage in first class is less likely. We are very sensitive to display our social status, and direct comparisons can lead to considerable social anxiety.

Both air rage, as well as income inequality, have increased during COVID-19. Yet media reporting this phenomenon consider more downstream—and individual—factors such as alcohol consumption, rather than class seating differences, as the cause.

Easily visible examples of social class differences abound in everyday life. Consider the businesses frequently seen in poorer parts of a city. A common sight is stores that advertise payday loans, with nail salons nearby. If you need money, you can borrow it, then go to a nearby nail salon where you can pay someone to sit below you, beautify your feet, and apply nail polish to reflect your higher status. Nail salons are an opportunity for those who lack the trappings of status to be pampered, to feel a momentary sense of entitlement. Someone else, likely an immigrant, is serving you, boosting your feeling of importance. You don't find payday loan stores and nail salons in wealthy neighborhoods.

Among rich countries, the proportion of the economy spent on advertising and marketing is associated with the income gap. The more inequality, the greater the percentage of the GDP spent on advertising. Where there is more equality the people in that society are less sensitive to advertising(27). Why?

Advertising primes us to buy goods. Shopping or retail therapy is a common but short-term way to cope with feelings brought about by inequality. Remember when you thought that buying just this one item would make you feel so much better? How long did that last? When I was working for an emergency department in the San Joaquin Valley of California one colleague was a keen photographer. When he arrived to spell me and do the next shift, I asked him how his day had been. He told me he had been sad so he purchased another camera. That made him feel better, but after a day the feeling was gone, and he was sad again. Acquiring more stuff only raises our mood for a brief period.

Inequality also leads to self-medicating with drugs. Three quarters of the world's opioid consumption takes place in the United States, where we have the highest rates of use. Opioid overdose death rates here have risen markedly since 1994, in contrast to those in other rich countries(28). Might the high use of opioids here reflect the increasing inequality and status anxiety? Studies show common forms of drug use, including opioids, cocaine, amphetamines, cannabis, and ecstasy, are higher in more unequal countries and more drug deaths occur in more unequal U.S. states.

Opioid use has soared in the United States during the COVID-19 pandemic. The increased stress people experiencing is exacerbated by the rising inequality. In 2020, drug overdose deaths in the United States rose to a record 93,000 which was 29% more than in 2019(29).

Illicit opioid use has tended to be concentrated among the poor, but rates are now increasing among middle-income Americans especially those who are White and have seen their status decline over the last decades. Increasing deaths among U.S. middle-aged Whites are termed "deaths of despair"(30). The less educated are very stressed and despondent about their future here. They often turn to alcohol, drugs of abuse, and suicide in their efforts to escape their terrifying downward spiral. A man in my West Seattle neighborhood faced eviction as the building in which he had his room was being sold. Unable to find any housing he could afford on his low disability checks, he ended his life by suicide.

Inequality also increases SARS-CoV-2 infection rates. Inequality increases distrust in institutions resulting in lower compliance with masking, quarantining, and immunizing. Poorer people in the United States are less likely to seek medical care and have more severe chronic diseases that increase infection risk. In Chapter 7, we will see that people lower down the socioeconomic ladder have weaker immune systems making them more susceptible to the virus.

A sense that "life is not fair" permeates discussions about the effects of inequality. This reaction can even be seen in other animals besides humans. Monkeys in lab settings are often rewarded for performing routine tasks with food such as a slice of a cucumber. They observe others doing the same task and getting the same reward. But when the reward is modified for one monkey, for example, by getting a grape instead of a slice of cucumber (the grape being the preferred food) for doing the same task, the monkey that doesn't get the grape becomes angry and agitated(31). These experiments have been repeated with other species including birds and dogs.

Do human beings naturally desire to be treated fairly like the monkeys described above? Like monkeys, we are primates. For most of human existence, hundreds of thousands of years, we lived as forager-hunters. Evidence points to these societies mostly practicing vigilant sharing and having sanctions against those who acted unfairly. Generally equality was the norm and gendered status differences small. We were innately altruistic, that is, we looked out for one another and were cooperative, fair, caring, and sharing. Where does selfishness come in? Evolution theory, beginning with Charles Darwin, posited both individual and group selection. Sociobiologists David Sloan Wilson and E.O. Wilson state, "Selfishness beats altruism within groups. Altruistic groups beat selfish groups." Within groups, there may be selfish individuals but groups who are inherently altruistic, that is, they look out for one another, will do better than those who are predominately selfish(32).

Social status and its psychological effects are comprehensively explored in *The Inner Level* by Wilkinson and Pickett(33).

All of these situations reflecting psychosocial status distinctions have biological consequences that affect our health that will be explored in Chapter 7.

We have thus far reviewed many ways in which our health is damaged by psychosocial factors, stress, and competition, that result from a large gap between rich and poor. Let's now consider Kawachi and Subramanian's third mechanism by which income inequality affects health.

Contextual or Pollution Effects

With a large income gap, the well-off pull away from the rest of society. Call it the secession of the rich. Consider the lifestyles of those on top of the unequal wealth distribution, the so-called one percent. They are actually the 0.1 or 0.01%. They live in gated communities, send their children to private schools, and have staff to clean their homes, do the gardening, and prepare meals. They enjoy private security services and receive concierge medical care from doctors and other service personnel who are at their beck and call. These very rich isolate themselves from the rest of society with their luxury yachts, private jets, and secluded islands in seeming paradises that we can't visit. They even used COVID-19 hideaways. Since they pay for these benefits with their high incomes, they don't see a need to support others who have considerably less. They often say, "We worked hard so that we can pay for these benefits ourselves why should we help others who didn't?" They essentially secede from the rest of society.

Most rich argue for less government intervention, less regulation, lower taxes, and letting the so-called free market dictate how society fares. While the rest of us work for wages or salaries, the rich get most of their income from what economists call rents or unearned income, for example, through investments in property or stocks—thus from means other than showing up at work. The inequality this system produces degrades the lives of others in society who work long, hard hours, doing unfulfilling work, sometimes at more than one job, just to make ends meet.

We are heading in the direction of even more concentrated political power, while the rest of us are facing an epidemic of disempowerment. Government funding for education decreases, the quality of public schools declines, and college students have to assume massive debt for an undergraduate degree. Public transportation and other social services are weakened. The deterioration in highway, bridge, and transportation systems, especially compared to other rich nations, shows the decline of infrastructure here. Stories of U.S. bridges and apartment buildings collapsing due to delayed maintenance or not heeding or delaying acting upon structural engineering reports are another example of the contextual effect of inequality. Access to healthcare is considered a privilege, not a fundamental human right as it is in many other nations. As the poor become disempowered and the wealthy gain power, societal relationships overall become less healthy.

During our COVID-19 catastrophe, more income inequality forces those with few savings to seek income doing risky essential work. These include elder and child care, cleaning services, transporting and delivering all the goods purchased online, and many others reflecting the inability to work from home. Those doing such work far from home face extended transportation issues with increased risk of viral transmission. Car sales have increased as those with financial means lessen the risk of becoming infected by avoiding public transport. At the same time, essential workers crowd together more increasing the risk of spread. There has been a push by those with wealth to move to rural areas with lower population density to lessen the risk of infection. Inequality is thus linked to increased COVID vulnerability, susceptibility, exposure, and transmission.

Social murder plays into the rise in COVID-19 deaths. Writing in 1847, Friedrich Engels described the condition of the working class in England where society was responsible for their suffering and dying younger than richer people. He called this murder as being the same as that with a lethal weapon. When politicians deny that there is a pandemic going on, or advocate allowing the infection to spread and support other policies that lead to non-COVID excess deaths, is this not murder? Another phrase for this process is structural violence, namely, how we create structures of inequality that lead to many more deaths than the behavioral kind. Social murder is the more descriptive—if not accurate—term(34). Political leaders have betrayed and killed their people.

U.S. President Obama said "inequality is the defining challenge of our time." But economic inequality has been with us at least since civilization. Civilization refers to a complex society characterized by social stratification and extreme inequality imposed by a cultural elite possessing a high degree of monopoly control over violence and ideology(35). Inequality is beholden to politics that generates an ideology where ordinary people defer to the views of elites and consider any change to lead to worse outcomes. This is very evident today where rising inequality is supported through the electoral process and the rise of strong men governments.

How Big Is Inequality in the United States?

Many ways can be used to describe inequality in a society. Mathematical formulas such as the Gini Index of Inequality are complicated to explain. Some have clever names such as the Robin Hood Index, which calculates how much would have to be redistributed to achieve equality. The proportion of people in the highest income range is another. Another common measure is the distribution of income among fifths, or quintiles, of the population. Studies demonstrate that most measures of inequality demonstrate similar impacts on health.

Another measure looks at the CEO employee-pay ratio, or how many times greater the income of the boss is compared to a rank and file worker in that organization. Such comparisons vary by industry, region of the country, and the size of the workforce and the corporation. In the 1950s, the ratio was around 10 or 20 to 1. For the last few years, publicly traded companies in the United States are required to disclose the CEO pay ratio. Figures today range up to more than 1000 to 1. The CEO in such a corporation makes a thousand times the pay of the company's median or middle worker which is a far cry from the situation in the early 1960s. In our COVIDian era, although there are signs that some CEO pay may be declining, the declines are greater among workers so that pay gap is increasing. In Japan, comparable figures are around 50 to 1.

According to the Forbes 2021 billionaire list, the wealth of Jeff Bezos, the richest person in the world, was 181 billion dollars. Elon Musk has now eclipsed that amount considerably. If we had freshly minted $100 bills (our largest currency denomination) and stacked one on top of another at sea level to total that wealth, the stack would reach 122 miles into space! In 2021, Bezos flew 62 miles into that space for ten minutes total ride time, reaching only about half of his wealth stack of $100 bills—while cutting the $2/hour hazard pay for Amazon workers working during the pandemic. But the pandemic was good to Bezos. His wealth increased *over 60 billion dollars in just one year* from 2019 to 2020. I am surprised at how few people in the United States are seething when presented with how much wealth a few people have. COVID-19 pandemic profiteering has increased inequality at a scale never seen before. Economic inequality is so extreme that the three richest people in the United States have more wealth than the bottom 160 million people here, while globally, billionaire wealth has more than doubled from 2019 to 2020, with one new billionaire added every 17 hours!

Since the global pandemic first hit, U.S. billionaires have grown $2 trillion dollars richer by October 2021(36). These new riches could finance much of the infrastructure and social spending legislation proposed by the Biden administration. Given our wealth hoarding system most of this new fortune will not be taxed and may disappear entirely through the efforts of the wealth defense industry(37).

Wealth, rather than income, is another way to make comparisons. A survey in 2005 asked Americans to estimate wealth distribution in the United States and to judge what was ideal(38). They were given three choices of wealth with one showing perfect equality, another showing the U.S. distribution of wealth (highly concentrated at the top) and a third being that of more equal Sweden. They were asked which distribution they would choose for themselves, also which reflected U.S. reality, and which they would choose if they had to be assigned to one of them. They mostly chose the two more equal ones as ideal for themselves or representing that of the United States. Americans vastly underestimate inequality in this country.

Despite underestimating inequality in our country, Americans' awareness of the problem is increasing. A 2020 Pew Research poll suggested 66% felt the federal government should have a large responsibility in reducing inequality with smaller proportions targeting large corporations and state governments with this task(39). Republicans are much less in favor of such efforts as they feel the rich work harder than others, while convincing those who are not rich that people with even less are the cause of their insecurity. Strong winds of change are blowing, something that hasn't been seen since the Great Depression. But as we found during the Great Depression, the impacts of poverty are far reaching, as we shall consider in the next chapter.

Other Effects of Inequality

Recently the United States has had a growing number of well-publicized mass shooting deaths. The media fan these flames, generating fear and moral panic. While the numbers affected are small compared to the excess deaths from other causes, they generate much public concern. Why are mass shootings increasing? A 2017 study by sociologists Roy Kwon and Joseph Cabrera implicated socio-structural factors. High county income inequality led to frustration, anger, and resentment leading to more such events. One outlet is to take it out on others through mass shootings. In a 2018 study, they found that counties with both high income inequality as well as high incomes create these environments, which result in such tragedies(40). A 2021 study by William Nugent and Anne Conway from the University of Tennessee showed that the rise in mass shootings over the last 54 years was correlated with our rise in income inequality(41). They found increasingly violent political rhetoric also increased mass shootings.

Robert Putnam's 2000 book *Bowling Alone* depicted the decline of social capital in the United States that was related to increasing economic inequality and led to increasing isolation(42). Social capital reflects the resources and benefits that individuals and groups acquire through connections with others, together with shared norms and values promoting cooperation measured in various ways. Social capital is the value we gain from our social networks—which enable us to access resources and opportunities. The rise of mass shootings reflects the decline of social capital here as communities have dispersed, industries that once supported whole families and communities have disappeared, and economic opportunities leading to upward social mobility declined while families fragmented geographically. Social capital also affects COVID-19 outcomes. More relational social capital, that is, stronger social connections within a community, resulted in lower deaths during the pandemic. Mechanisms include following pandemic guidelines, such as masking, physical distancing, and vaccination, to avoid SARS-CoV-2 infection.

Economic inequality affects rates of homicides in most countries(43). This association is evident among U.S. states, where those with more unequal income distributions have considerably more homicides—over five times higher than in the most equal states. Poverty doesn't explain this trend. Firearm availability is also a factor, but economic inequality matters more when considering all factors together. Younger men, who have more of a taste for risk, do most of the killing. Today the stress of living with so much inequality is reflected in outbursts of violence. Young men are typical victims as well as the perpetrators. Such people, when under extreme stress, compete with similar others to kill their competitors.

To put homicide into perspective, a number of countries have higher rates than that of the United States. Some American cities, however, such as New Orleans and Chicago, have murder rates that are comparable to those of high-poverty, high-homicide nations such as Honduras and South Africa. And while there are other countries with higher homicide rates, the United States has the highest homicide rate among rich nations. Such violence seems a fabric of life in this country. During the COVID-19 pandemic, homicide rates have increased in U.S. cities. The rising inequality, which leads to putting down those below you, often permanently into the grave, as described above, is hard at work in America.

A range of medical conditions are linked to inequality. Heart failure, a common chronic disease where the cardiac system is unable to adequately pump blood to major organs like the lungs and brain, is more common where there is more income inequality. A study of over 15,000 patients in 54 countries looked at hospitalization, cardiovascular death, and overall mortality from that disease(44). After statistically adjusting for various factors to attenuate the effect of income inequality, it remained an important predictor of worse mortality outcomes. Increased chronic stress leads to biological changes that are known to affect heart health. Broader social and structural mechanisms that were identified as relevant included lower levels of social capital in more unequal countries, lower rates of social service spending, and fewer safety nets. The political decisions that lead to these factors exemplify social murder.

The recent #MeToo response to long-standing sexual abuse by those with status reflects decreased tolerance of inequality in a patriarchal society, where men command seemingly absolute power and enough money to harass others at will. Some have termed this "fuck you" money, that is, the amount of money you need to do what you want. Until recently, the rich and powerful could do whatever they wanted to women without fear of repercussions. Many people, mostly men, crave this power, and for decades they were protected by underlings from the abuse coming to light. People such as Bill Cosby, Harvey Weinstein, and Jeffrey Epstein had public or media personae entirely opposite to their behaviors in real life. Although a few men in exalted status positions are being dethroned, some of them were paid millions of dollars in bonuses when they lost their jobs. Other abusers may return to harass. Some, such as Donald Trump, are thus far immune to prosecution for such allegations.

The increasing attention paid to sexual harassment, rape, and other forms of violence toward women reflects an awareness of gender inequality in society. Intimate partner violence (IPV) is the commonest form of violence toward women globally. I would often see battered women in the emergency department. After treating them I would try to get them into shelters anonymously to be safe for at least a while. Most women would not comply. Given the reluctance of many people to report it, and the challenges in documenting it accurately, IPV is difficult to study and even to report.

What level of inequality should we aim for? Almost 2500 years ago, Plato wrote,

> The form of law which I should propose as the natural sequel would be as follows: In a state which is desirous of being saved from all plagues—not fact but rather distraction—there should exist among the citizens neither extreme poverty, nor, again, excess of wealth, for both are productive of these evils. Now the legislator should determine what is to be the limit of poverty or wealth. Let the limit of poverty be the value of the lot; this ought to be preserved, and no rule, nor any one else who aspires after a reputation for virtue, will allow the lot to be impaired in any case. This the legislator gives as a measure, and he will permit a man to acquire double or triple, or as much as four times the amount of this.

In other words, Plato would limit the income or wealth gap to be no more than four to one(45). Today's gap is on the order of two hundred billion to one!

Criticisms of the Inequality-Health Relationship

Why is inequality strongly linked to so many adverse health and social outcomes? To some it may be intuitive, but a common contrary view is that inequality is what makes us better people. Isn't striving, overcoming obstacles, pulling ourselves up by our bootstraps what makes America great? That argument presupposes that those who are on the lower social rungs do not strive, have not overcome obstacles, and have not pulled themselves up by the bootstraps—and that those who are perched on the upper rungs have.

Arguments that inequality is good for us have looked at materialist explanations, such as the view that with a big gap between rich and poor, the rich can purchase more "stuff" that improves not only their well-being but that of the rest of us who produce this "stuff." That argument is based on the trickle-down theory that the wealthy do spend their money, when in fact, most of it is invested in intangible investments such as stocks which disproportionately advantage other wealthy people. Moreover, as production is moved overseas, where wages are lower, fewer workers in America will benefit from the purchases of the wealthy. Only recently has it been more widely recognized that inequality does not improve economies and is a deeply damaging social force, at the root of many if not most of our national ills.

After *The Spirit Level* was published in 2009 many critical comments appeared including titles such as *Beware False Prophets: Equality, the Good*

Society and The Spirit Level as well as *Spirit Level Delusion: Fact-Checking the Left's New Theory of Everything* both in 2010. Wilkinson and Pickett responded with a 2011 revised edition of *The Spirit Level* that addressed the critics. In the ensuing decade criticisms continue to appear that are minor and help elucidate nuances. In *Social Science and Medicine,* Simone Rambotti, a sociologist at the University of Arizona, questioned the relationship between inequality and poverty in 2015. This was followed by Pickett and Wilkinson's response and then Rambotti's rejoinder which focused on small points of epidemiologic analysis(46). I consider these healthy criticisms. Recent studies refine the inequality health relationship by, for example, decomposing it through four age ranges for COVID deaths among 22 countries. As had previously been shown, inequality kills more younger people than older ones from COVID.

While income inequality is a direct health hazard, rapid changes in income inequality can produce accelerated health effects. Let's consider some examples of natural experiments. Income inequality can decrease rapidly, as happened in Japan after World War II and in China after the 1949 revolution. Dramatic health improvements were seen in both countries in the ensuing decade. By 1978, Japan had become the longest-lived country in the world. We will explore reasons for Japan's good health in Chapter 8. China in the 1950s had dramatic decreases in child mortality when inequality did not rise(47). With the reforms starting around 1980, the improvements were more modest.

More gradual decreases in income inequality may produce slower improvements in health. After the economic depression that began in 1929, inequality decreased and health improved, so that by the early 1950s the United States was one of the world's healthiest countries. After the 1970s, as the manufacturing base shifted from the United States to other nations where wages were lower, wages for low-skilled workers here plummeted. Inequality increased, and the U.S. health advantage was lost.

After the Soviet Union collapsed in 1991, income and wealth inequality skyrocketed in many of the republics. Suddenly state assets were commandeered by oligarchs. Russia experienced a rapid health decline, with mortality increasing dramatically in both men and women(48). It has taken almost 30 years for health to return to pre-breakup levels there.

Social murder killed those in many countries of the former Soviet Union. Suddenly, massive inequality was imposed, but the violence was invisible. People were dying of the usual causes, heart disease and others, exacerbated by stress that resulted in considerably increased consumption of alcohol, especially by single, middle-aged men(49). There was no smoking gun. Social murder was the physical and psychological harm resulting from exploitative and unjust social, political, and economic systems.

COVID-19 deaths in the United States represent social murder. When the virus spread government policies ignored and downplayed the threat, and discouraged preventive measures such as wearing masks, distancing, and getting tested, leading to the most deaths of any country in 2020. Whether you call it structural violence or social murder, such suffering results from the lack of political attention paid to the social determinants of health—a concept we will explore in Chapter 6. Concurrent with the rapid rise of income and wealth inequality in the United States, our life expectancy and other mortality measures have worsened considerably. Although it is too early to be certain, we may be experiencing the impact of abruptly increasing inequality leading to marked rises in mortality that may take a long time to reverse as Russia demonstrates.

Conclusion

Economic inequality, either in income or wealth, has no good features. Many books and treatises make this point. Is inequality's effect on health an open-and-shut case? Yes, Jan Vandenmoortele concludes that inequality has a deep and far-reaching influence on people and society, engendering near universal harm(50). Consider the movement to ban nuclear weapons that began in earnest in the 1950s when it was clear that humanity would not survive a nuclear war and there was no reason to have such armaments. That recognition didn't stop quite a few countries from maintaining a nuclear arsenal. But few of us think nuking others is a viable strategy for solving our problems. Economic inequality is the equivalent of a nuclear weapon. Its impact on the population is devastating and deadly.

We began this chapter by heading upstream to understand why so many people catapulted down the swift river and required rescue at great cost. The steep slope that led to people falling into the river mirrors the profound effect of our vast income inequality. It produces a fog of psychosocial stress that limits the cooperative relationships needed for good health. We are not schooled to look at fundamental causes for problems that range beyond what we can do individually to change. The political system that produces our vast economic inequality seems far removed from what produces our own health. In order to address those major impediments, we must look at the foundational mechanisms that link inequality to worse health. We must turn to inequality's sibling, poverty, and ask, how did poverty come into being and what does it have to do with our health?

Questions to Consider and Discuss

1. Many Americans appear to have little interest in decreasing inequality despite the extreme levels present today. Why? How do you feel about the issue?
2. What ways exist to highlight the pivotal importance of economic inequality impacting health?

References

1. Wilkinson RG. Income Distribution and Life Expectancy. BMJ. 1992;304(6820):165–8.
2. Kaplan GA, Pamuk ER, Lynch JW, Cohen RD, Balfour JL. Inequality in Income and Mortality in the United States: Analysis of Mortality and Potential Pathways. BMJ. 1996; 312(7037):999–1003.
3. Kennedy BP, Kawachi I, Prothrow SD. Income Distribution and Mortality: Cross Sectional Ecological Study of the Robin Hood index in the United States. BMJ. 1996; 312(7037):1004–7.
4. Lynch JW, Kaplan GA, Pamuk ER, Cohen RD, Heck KE, Balfour JL, et al. Income Inequality and Mortality in Metropolitan Areas of the United States. American Journal of Public Health. 1998;88:1074–80.
5. Wilkinson RG. Unhealthy Societies: The Afflictions of Inequality. London: Routledge; 1996.
6. Oronce CIA, Scannell CA, Kawachi I, Tsugawa Y. Association Between State-Level Income Inequality and COVID-19 Cases and Mortality in the USA. Journal of General Internal Medicine. 2020;35(9):2791–3.
7. Tan AX, Hinman JA, Abdel Magid HS, Nelson LM, Odden MC. Association Between Income Inequality and County-Level COVID-19 Cases and Deaths in the US. JAMA Network Open. 2021;4(5):e218799.
8. Elgar FJ, Stefaniak A, Wohl MJA. The Trouble With Trust: Time-Series Analysis of Social Capital, Income Inequality, and COVID-19 Deaths in 84 Countries. Social Science & Medicine. 2020;263:113365.
9. Surgeon General. Smoking and Health: Report of the Advisory Committee to the Surgeon General of the Public Health Service. Washington, DC: US Department of Health, Education and Welfare; 1964.
10. Pickett KE, Wilkinson RG. Income Inequality and Health: A Causal Review. Social Science & Medicine. 2015;128(0):316–26.
11. Miller JD, Scott EC, Okamoto S. Public Acceptance of Evolution. Science. 2006;313(5788):765–6.
12. Wilkinson R, Pickett KE. The Spirit Level: Why Greater Equality Makes Societies Stronger. New York, NY: Bloomsbury; 2011.
13. Kawachi I, Subramanian S. Income Inequality. In: Berkman LF, Kawachi I, Glymour MM, editors. Social Epidemiology. New York, NY: Oxford University Press; 2014. p. 126–51.
14. Fiske ST. Envy up, Scorn Down: How Comparison Divides Us. American Psychologist. 2010;65(8):698–706.
15. Shaw GB. The Intelligent Woman's Guide to Socialism and Capitalism. New York, NY: Brentano's; 1928.
16. Sherman R. Uneasy street: the Anxieties of Affluence. Princeton: Princeton University Press; 2017.
17. Layte R, Whelan CT. Who Feels Inferior? A Test of the Status Anxiety Hypothesis of Social Inequalities in Health. European Sociological Review. 2014;30(4):525–35.
18. Marmot M. Status Syndrome - How Our Position on the Social Gradient Affects Longevity and Health. London: Bloomsbury; 2004.
19. Singh-Manoux A, Adler NE, Marmot MG. Subjective Social Status: Its Determinants and Its Association With Measures of Ill-Health in the Whitehall II Study. Social Science & Medicine. 2003;56(6):1321–33.

20. Sapolsky RM. Social Status and Health in Humans and Other Animals. Annual Review of Anthropology. 2004;33(1):393–418.

21. Marx K, Engels F. The Communist Manifesto: a Road Map to History's Most Important Political Document. In: Gasper P, editor. Chicago, Ill: Haymarket Books; 2005.

22. Piff PK, Stancato DM, Mendoza-Denton R, Keltner D, Coteb S. Higher Social Class Predicts Increased Unethical Behavior. Proceedings of the National Academy of Sciences of the United States of America. 2012;109(11):4086–91.

23. Imam SZ, Karanasios G, Khatib M, Cavale N, Amar O, Mayou B. Resumption of Cosmetic Surgery During COVID – Experience of a Specialised Cosmetic Surgery Day-Case Hospital. Journal of Plastic, Reconstructive & Aesthetic Surgery. 2021;74(11):3178–85.

24. Smith A. The Theory of Moral Sentiments. London: A. Millar and A. Kincaid and J. Bell; 1759.

25. Solnick SJ, Hemenway D. Is More Always Better?: A Survey on Positional Concerns. Journal of Economic Behavior & Organization. 1998;37(3):373–83.

26. McLinton SS, Drury D, Masocha S, Savelsberg H, Martin L, Lushington K. "Air Rage": A Systematic Review of Research on Disruptive Airline Passenger Behaviour 1985-2020. Journal of Airline and Airport Management. 2020;10(1):31–49.

27. Wilkinson RG, Pickett KE. The Enemy between Us: The Psychological and Social Costs of Inequality. European Journal of Social Psychology. 2017;47(1):11–24.

28. Ho JY. The Contemporary American Drug Overdose Epidemic in International Perspective. Population and Development Review. 2019;45(1):7–40.

29. Katz J, Sanger-Katz M. "It's Huge, It's Historic, It's Unheard-of": Drug Overdose Deaths Spike New York: New York Times; 2021 [cited 2021 July 14]. Available from: https://www.nytimes.com/interactive/2021/07/14/upshot/drug-overdose-deaths.html.

30. Case A, Deaton A. Deaths of Despair and the Future of Capitalism. Princeton: Princeton University Press; 2020.

31. Brosnan SF, De Waal FB. Monkeys Reject Unequal Pay. Nature. 2003;425(6955):297–9.

32. Wilson DS, Wilson EO. Rethinking the Theoretical Foundation of Sociobiology. The Quarterly Review of Biology. 2007;82(4):327–48.

33. Wilkinson R, Pickett K. The Inner Level: How More Equal Societies Reduce Stress, Restore Sanity and Improve Everybody's Well-Being. New York, NY: Penguin; 2019.

34. Medvedyuk S, Govender P, Raphael D. The Reemergence of Engels' Concept of Social Murder in Response to Growing Social and Health Inequalities. Social Science & Medicine. 2021;289:114377.

35. Wisman, J.D. The Origins and Dynamics of Inequality : Sex, Politics, and Ideology. New York, NY: Oxford University Press; 2022.

36. Collins C. Updates: Billionaire Wealth, U.S. Job Losses and Pandemic Profiteers Washington, D.C.: Institute for Policy Studies; 2021 [cited 2021 October 18]. Available from: https://inequality.org/great-divide/updates-billionaire-pandemic/?emci=b55c3deb-2e30-ec11-981f-c896653b9208&emdi=b302e29f-4530-ec11-981f-c896653b9208&ceid=4064139.

37. Collins C. The Wealth Hoarders: How Billionaires Pay Millions to Hide Trillions. Cambridge, UK: Polity; 2021.

38. Norton MI, Ariely D. Building a Better America-One Wealth Quintile at a Time. Perspectives on Psychological Science. 2011;6(1):9–12.

39. Horowitz JM, Igielnik R, Kochhar R. Views on Reducing Economic Inequality. Washington, D.C.: Pew Research Center; 2020 [cited 2020 January 9]. Available from: https://www.pewresearch.org/social-trends/2020/01/09/views-on-reducing-economic-inequality/.

40. Cabrera JF, Kwon R. Income Inequality, Household Income, and Mass Shooting in the United States. Frontiers in Public Health. 2018 Oct 17;6:294.

41. Nugent WR, Conway A. Violent Political Rhetoric, Generalized Imitation, Income Inequality, Gun Ownership, Changes in Gross Domestic Product, and Mass Shootings. Journal of Social Service Research. 2021;47(5):694–713.

42. Putnam RD. Bowling Alone: The Collapse and Revival of American Community. New York, NY: Simon and Schuster; 2000.

43. Daly M. Killing the Competition: Economic Inequality and Homicide. New Brunswick: Transaction Publishers; 2016.

44. Dewan P, Rørth R, Jhund PS, Ferreira JP, Zannad F, Shen L, et al. Income Inequality and Outcomes in Heart Failure: A Global Between-Country Analysis. JACC: Heart Failure. 2019;7(4):336–46.

45. Plato. Inequality in the Distribution of Wealth. The Dialogues of Plato. IV. Oxford: Clarendon Press; 1953. pp. 313–4.

46. Pickett KE, Wilkinson RG. Recalibrating Rambotti: Disentangling Concepts of Poverty and Inequality. Social Science & Medicine. 2015;139:132–4.

47. Babiarz KS, Eggleston K, Miller G, Zhang Q. An Exploration of China's Mortality Decline Under Mao: A Provincial Analysis, 1950–80. Population Studies. 2015;69(1):39–56.

48. Marmot M, Bobak M. International Comparators and Poverty and Health in Europe. BMJ. 2000;321(7269):1124–8.

49. Parsons MA. Dying Unneeded: The Cultural Context of the Russian Mortality Crisis. Nashville: Vanberbilt University Press; 2014.

50. Vandemoortele J. The Open-and-Shut Case Against Inequality. Development Policy Review. 2021;39(1):135–51.

Chapter 4

Poverty Perspectives

I've been rich and I've been poor and rich is better.

Attributed to the siren Mae West (and others)

Being poor is bad for your health. Bill Foege, a key player in eradicating smallpox and later the head of the CDC, wrote in his book *The Fears of The Rich, The Needs of The Poor: My Years at the CDC,*

> The current corollary to slavery is poverty….It is the single most impor-
> tant determinant of health. It is not just that poor people have poor
> health. Various studies have shown that the healthiest societies are those
> with the narrowest income inequality gap. Poverty breeds discontent, and
> the poor often attempt through crime or social disruption to remedy the
> disparities. Michael Manley, formerly the Prime Minister of Jamaica, once
> said that, "Poverty shared can be endured." Modern communications have
> demonstrated to the poor around the world that their condition is not
> being shared.(1)

Being poor shortens your life. Those who have been poor would not recom-
mend it. Michael Marmot, a leading figure on population health, writing in
The Status Syndrome, describes a cruel joke about poverty(2). "The bad news is
that it makes you miserable, the good news is that you won't have to survive
it for too long." As on target as his joke might be, the question for us is, what
would it take to make poverty more survivable?

Invention of Poverty

One might believe the biblical invocation that the poor will always be with
us. But is that true? Is being poor a part of human existence? Anatomically
modern humans have been around for perhaps half a million years. For more
than 99 percent of that time, the Paleolithic, we lived as forager-hunters with
other societal arrangements.

DOI: 10.4324/9781003315889-5

The neuroscientist Robert Sapolsky whom we met in the previous chapter in defining poverty writes,

> ... and in many ways it was one of the great stupid moves of all time. Hunter-gatherers have thousands of wild sources of food to subsist on. Agriculture changed all that, generating an overwhelming reliance on a few dozen domesticated food sources, making you extremely vulnerable to the next famine, the next locust infestation, the next potato blight. Agriculture allowed for the stockpiling of surplus resources and thus, inevitably, the unequal stockpiling of them—stratification of society and the invention of classes. Thus, it allowed for the invention of poverty. I think that the punch line of the primate-human difference is that when humans invented poverty, they came up with a way of subjugating the low-ranking like nothing ever before seen in the primate world.(3)

Poverty wasn't present for most of human existence. In the Paleolithic, we lived in pristine environments that sustained us with wide varieties of plant and animal foods. Archaeologists find little evidence of Paleolithic famines and few signs of nutritional deficiencies on these ancient bones. Anthropologist Marshall Sahlins, writing about the stone age, said, "The world's most primitive people have few possessions, but they are not poor. Poverty is not a certain small amount of goods, nor is it just a relation between means and ends; above all it is a relation between people. Poverty is a social status. As such it is an invention of civilization. It has grown with civilization ... as an invidious distinction between classes."(4)

The Jewish origins story in Genesis of the Old Testament says Adam and Eve were cast out of the Garden of Eden and given seeds to grow their food. Yet, the notion that humans have planted their food since our species' origins is a myth. Agriculture tended to be adopted by necessity, due to increasing population size and decreasing food availability. Forager-hunters resisted adopting agriculture for as long as possible because they were able to subsist on what they could gather and hunt, usually without much work. They likely practiced vigilant sharing, as modern forger-hunters do today. Those who try to become authoritarian by not sharing equitably would be criticized, ridiculed, ostracized, or, if necessary, executed. Such practices were required to survive as a society and continue today, because to deny someone sufficient food can potentially be a death sentence(5, 6).

With the adoption of agriculture, however, diets became more monotonous. Farmers grew only a few crops, then harvested them, while planting the next crops, and so on through the seasons. This required an enormous amount of physical labor in contrast to the forager-hunter epoch where mostly women gathered foods for a few hours a day, and every few weeks, the men went off on a hunt. They were the original leisure time society. Moreover, forager-hunters were not stationary, as later agriculturalists became. They moved to where food was plentiful, enabling wild habitats to regenerate so their environment continued to sustain them. Many former concepts of the forager-hunter era are being updated to show that they did not progress linearly to the adoption of modern forms of life, but in the Epipaleolithic, they experimented with various ways of forming societies that included hierarchies, class divisions, specialization, occasional farming, and seasonal settlements(5, 7). There is much to be learned about Paleolithic societies, but today's concept of poverty was mostly absent then.

Contrary to the popular opinion of progress, health declined with the advent of agriculture. Reasons include poor nutrition, famines, stress, and increased exposure to infectious diseases by living close to domesticated animals or by destroying wild animal habitats(8). Tuberculosis came from bovines as did cowpox and smallpox, flu from domestic fowl and pigs, measles from cattle farming in the Middle East, and, more recently, HIV from non-human primates and SARS from bats.

Once food such as grains could be stored or livestock kept in fenced pastures, someone could amass great stores and declare themselves Lord or Master. They could tell others to produce food for the "Master," build a castle in which to store it, and go to war to defend his wealth. The planting, harvesting, storing, and distributing of food generally produced substantial hierarchies.

Stationary settlements began, and craft specialization developed. With the emergence of villages and towns came private property. Then civilizations, which can be considered as complex societies characterized by urban development, social stratification, and extreme inequality imposed by a cultural elite possessing a high degree of monopoly control over violence and ideology(9). This shift led to power relationships, including the subordination of women as men became warriors, and property was conferred upon males as reward for their service. At the same time, transmittable diseases soared as populations became more concentrated.

With the advent of agriculture, life expectancy declined and infant mortality increased(10). Natural birth control with long durations of breastfeeding declined as early weaning foods became available, thus increasing women's fertility. At the same time, women's labor increased as they planted, weeded, and harvested the fields and did most of the domestic work as well, with cultivated foods taking much longer to prepare than food gathered from the wilds. The result was that women's labor increased much more than men's, and such labor differences continue today.

Our health, as estimated by mortality rates, has only begun to improve in the last century or two. Taking stature (adult height) as a measure of health, the overall trend until recently has been downward or at least not increasing. Anthropologist Mark Nathan Cohen writes, "The seventeenth- and eighteenth-century Europeans against whom we proudly measure ourselves to demonstrate our progress, were actually some of the smallest people who ever lived."(11)

A close look at the armor of British leaders in the Tower of London demonstrates his point. Soldiers of the past were not very tall. Another proxy measure is the notably short grave boxes in old English cathedrals, demonstrating how much smaller the British used to be in the past.

Although recognizing poverty's broader effects would take millennia, the impacts of rising social hierarchies were apparent early on. Thus, we might ask, why would poverty have been invented when it made health decline and did not even benefit those who were not poor? Sapolsky suggests it was to subjugate the low ranking. That is, even though as a group, populations had poorer health through agriculture, because agriculture enabled a minority to control food resources, it was able to keep the poor in their place and not let them get any ideas of overthrowing the rich and powerful—a perception of material resources and status differences which remains true to this day. Consider the many ways the poor are put down today.

Making the poor feel inferior on account of social stratification allowed various forms of control such as slavery, which mostly arose with the rise of civilizations some 5000 years ago. The transatlantic slave trade began with the first arrival of West Africans to the New World said to be in 1619 and significantly expanded the enslavement of people and conferred on the institution of slavery a racial dimension that had previously been absent. Although slavery is now illegal worldwide, various forms of human trafficking, including bonded labor, forced child labor, and sex trafficking, continue—something that was unheard of before the rise of agriculture and only became possible when humans shifted from egalitarian societies to hierarchical ones.

Consider poverty and inequality then as siblings that come from the same national parent and have been birthed by the technological advances that facilitated the rise in agriculture and thus civilization. While we may have made great strides in reducing slavery throughout the world, caste or class systems[1] persist to keep certain sectors of the population in power, and others from becoming powerful.

Measuring and Defining Poverty

There are no uniform measures across the world to count the poor. The World Bank uses an international poverty line, a daily income amount, to describe those in extreme poverty. Originally, it was set at a dollar a day (in purchasing power parity) in 1985 and has been raised since. In 2017, the daily income below which someone was considered impoverished was $1.90 a day with almost ten percent of people around the world falling below that level. Just four years later, in 2021, that number has increased due to the pandemic which has left even more people in extreme poverty—reflecting an unprecedented increase.

In urban, industrial countries, poverty looks very different than it does in rural developing countries which tend to have stronger kinship networks providing safety nets for those with insufficient resources. In its 1979

Supplemental Benefits Commission report, the British government described poverty as a standard of living so low that it excludes and isolates people from the rest of the community(12). "To keep out of poverty, people must have an income which enables them to participate in society. For example, they must be able to keep themselves reasonably fed and dressed well enough to maintain their self-respect and to attend interviews for jobs with confidence. Their homes must be reasonably warm; their children should not feel shamed by the quality of their clothing; the family must be able to visit relatives, and give them something for birthdays and Christmas; they must be able to read newspapers[2] and maintain their membership of trade unions and churches. They must be able to live in a way which ensures, so far as possible, that public officials, doctors, teachers, landlords, and others treat them with the courtesy due to every member of the community." Similarly, the Council of European Communities defined poverty as the "individuals or families whose resources are so small as to exclude them from the minimum acceptable way of life of the Member State in which they live." In this way, poverty is not defined in terms of low income or few resources, but rather is conceived as social standing relative to the rest of society.

Relative poverty measures are commonly used to provide a more accurate assessment of poverty. In the United Kingdom today, households are considered poor if their income is 60% below the median (middle) household income after adjusting for housing costs for that year. Similar relative household income measures are used in other European nations. The United States uses an absolute measure for an individual with daily income less than $36, or for a family of four with less than $72. The official poverty measure here is set at a pretax cash income of three times the cost of a minimum food diet in 1963 and adjusted for family size. Relative poverty measures are more impacted by income inequality than absolute ones. Using the relative measure for the United States, poverty is about double that of the United Kingdom(13). The focus on impacting poverty in the United Kingdom considers providing a safety net, while in the United States, there are piecemeal supplements such as food stamps. The flawed U.S. measure is supplemented (but not replaced) by a more complicated Supplemental Poverty Measure including more factors.

Depending on who you consider rich nations to be, the United States has the distinction of being second only to Mexico in having the most poverty and the most child poverty of any rich nation(14).

Being Poor in Different Countries

Poverty or being poor has different connotations around the world. So-called poor laws were adopted in parts of Western Europe a few hundred years ago to distinguish those who were lazy from those more deserving. Such laws gave governments the ability to raise taxes and maintain so-called almshouses to provide indoor relief for the aged, handicapped, and other worthy poor. Paupers were also dependent on various charities. In England, these policies continued until after World War II when the modern welfare state was created. Forms patterned on the English poor law model were variously used in the colonies that became the United States.

In Sweden, poor laws were organized by the church in the 1600s and nationalized in 1847. Benefits were initially largely restricted to orphans, the aged, and invalids. In the 20th century, these practices transformed into their modern social welfare system.

American poor laws provide relief through state mechanisms that vary tremendously. In the United States, the Great Depression fostered the federal New Deal legislation, which provided social security benefits, unemployment insurance, jobs programs, and a minimum wage and was the first major step in dealing with poverty. The ethic of the undeserving poor continues to be a major impediment to dealing with poverty in the United States.

Even when benefits are available, such as the Earned Income Tax Credit, which provides poor families with a tax credit of a few thousand dollars, they can receive even if they owe no taxes, perhaps a fifth don't claim this assistance, perhaps because they do not know about it. Poorer people also may not use such tax credits in the United States because of difficulties in filling out the forms. For others, accepting government assistance is an admission that they couldn't do it on their own. They would have to confess failure in our meritocracy.

The prevailing belief regarding why poor people are poor varies among nations. A World Values Survey found that the largest proportion, about half of Americans, say the reason adults are poor is because such people are lazy or lack will power. In Norway, more than half say that people are poor due to injustices in society(15).

President Johnson's "War on Poverty" declaration in 1964 produced legislation expanding social security, and other benefits that had limited impacts on the poor. In the United States, many believe that the poor should be punished for being poor, a steadily growing belief since President Clinton's 1996 Welfare Reform. That legislation gave states the right to set their own rules for assistance and imposed lifetime five year limits on benefits. We also began locking the poor up in prisons. This practice accelerated significantly with the rise of the "War on Drugs," which had a much greater impact on the poor and people of color than it did on wealthier drug users. We now house a quarter of the world's prisoners in the United States, with almost one in a hundred Americans behind bars(16).

We not only lock up our poor, we are the only developed nation which funds its public schools based on property taxes, which ensures that people growing up in poor areas will go to schools receiving the least funding. Other rich nations fund schools through overall budgets. We have created a system where wealthier students are tracked to college and poor students are tracked to menial jobs that don't pay enough to live on—giving rise to crime and drug addiction, and no access to treatment for dependency. As a result, these students grow up in what is essentially a school to prison pipeline.

Mark Twain captured the absurdity of our school to prison pipeline when he wrote, "When I was a boy on the Mississippi River there was a proposition in a township there to discontinue public schools because they were too expensive. An old farmer spoke up and said if they stopped building the schools they would not save anything, because every time a school was closed a jail had to be built."

Today, despite all our prosperity, many Americans live in extreme squalor lacking plumbing, electricity, and safe shelter. Over half a million U.S. households lack indoor plumbing. Where I live in Seattle, the rise of Amazon, Microsoft, and other industries brought high-paying jobs to the city. Unfortunately, as a result of those high-paying jobs, housing costs increased so much that affordable housing is all but gone. The freeways and downtown streets are now lined by tents where the unhoused live year round. While many citizens rage against their presence, they vote against investing in their housing.

Despite our failure to help our poor, there are many structures in place to assist us in other ways that we take for granted. Consider handrails on stairs that are required by building codes, or smoke detectors and fire sprinklers found in public places or street lighting required in residential neighborhoods. These are safeguards for our physical safety, yet few of these structural assists are targeted specifically for the poor.

Poverty is a serious disability—an impairment that profoundly affects a person's life in many ways. Wheelchair users get ramps built on sidewalks and other assistance for mobility, the blind get Braille buttons on elevators, and the hearing-impaired get sign language on visual performances. But housing, heating, sanitation, transportation, or internet access for the poor are not given similar recognition as basic human needs. We must eliminate poverty, as the fundamental American disability. Instead of making progress on how we support the poor, their support has been increasingly eroded and will become worse in coming years.

Health Improvements in the Last Few Centuries

Declines in mortality occurred in most parts of the world during the last century. But increases were seen with the 1918 Influenza Pandemic as well as both world wars. Since the 1950s, our mortality has increasingly lagged behind other countries, both rich and poorer. The gap between life expectancies among all countries has decreased from about 37 years in the early 1990s to 32 years in 2019, but COVID has increased it. Some countries which dealt with the virus early on have seen fewer deaths, and those that did not, such as the United States, have seen far more deaths.

Progress in reducing poverty and raising the standard of living accounts for much of the global gains in life expectancy. More of the improvements came from reducing mortality among younger people. Infant and child mortality reductions had a big effect. In the 18th and 19th centuries, available studies in some European cities show how those in the lowest social strata had as much as five times higher risk of dying. Reducing the squalor in urban areas made a big difference in decreasing mortality amongst the poor. Social and economic improvements produced health gains. Fostering a better early life, as we shall see in the next chapter, has also had a big impact.

Poverty Issues

Though I generally do not take a disease perspective in this book, examples of heart disease, lung disease, and others creep in during our quest to understand various health concepts. Poorer people, in general, are more likely to suffer from various diseases and tend to respond less well to treatments compared to richer patients.

Dr. Samuel Broder, the director of the National Cancer Institute in 1989, said *"poverty is a carcinogen."* Poorer people, who politically have much less power than wealthier folk, are more likely to live in unhealthy environments and be exposed to cancer-causing agents. When the poor get cancer, they are less likely to get good treatment and to survive(17). Since cancers, like most diseases, have a predilection for worse outcomes among the poor, this analogy should not be surprising. There is something about being poor that predisposes you to having poor outcomes from cancer conditions, as Broder implied. Overall death rates from cancer are higher for the poor than they are for the wealthy. If all people aged 25–64 had the same cancer death rates as the most highly educated White Americans, there would be a third fewer deaths in the United States from cancer every year.[3]

Is it possible to be "rich" or affluent without material wealth or abundance? Recall my experiences in Nepal in Chapter 3, a very poor country both then and now. In the mid-1970s, I lived in Dhorpatan, a week's walk from the road where I helped set up a community health project. This was a region of subsistence agriculture that was isolated from the forces of materialism. The people I lived among exhibited self-respect. They appeared satisfied with their lives; though they had little, they had the necessities of life and strong social ties. In those earlier years, I never heard Nepali people speak of themselves as poor. But as economic development spread, bringing roads, electricity, and eventually the internet, concepts of poverty entered the discourse. Close to the road, people began to talk of being poor. Once, not far from the road, I walked along the trail with a young student who was practicing his English. "Nepal is a very poor country," he said. I asked in Nepali how he came to know this. "I learned it in my English class at school," he replied. I came to see that economic development teaches people to be poor. In the 1990s, when evaluating child survival projects funded by the U.S. government, I learned some people were taught to call themselves "the poorest of the poor." Imagine trying to live with that label!

To be poor in a wealthy society can be the worst form of poverty. As I noted in Chapter 3, if everyone was poor, no one would be. Well, the same can be said of wealth. If everyone was rich, no one would be. Those who are affluent require that there be poor to know they are rich. As a poor person in the United States, you may have a smartphone, perhaps a small apartment, and a menial job in a fast food establishment earning minimum wage. But you are surrounded by the trappings of wealth, and may blame yourself for not having worked harder and gotten further ahead in life. You may manage by self-medicating with drugs to get through the day, by smoking, drinking, or by eating comfort foods—foods high in carbohydrates, sugars, fats, and salts. These coping mechanisms lead to worse health.

Most people characterized as poor in the United States don't call themselves poor, however. Poor people in the United States call themselves broke, homeless, temporarily unemployed, or having a cash flow problem, but they are unlikely to call themselves poor. To admit you are poor means you will never strike it rich and achieve the American Dream. The American Dream in the United States is about being able to become wealthy through hard work and perseverance. The rags to riches transformation is perceived of as not only possible, but probable. That possibility was much more achievable in the middle of the last century than at present. Income or social advancement in the United States is now considerably less than it was even a few decades ago. Upward economic mobility is greater now in most other rich nations. Many people on the lower end of the hierarchy in the United States feel stuck and despair about ever being able to move up. Still, a remarkable percentage of the public believes that before they die, they will be rich. Although it is a nightmare, if you are asleep, you can experience the American Dream.

One study compared attitudes toward their own upward mobility among people in the United States, France, Italy, Sweden, and the United Kingdom(18). When considering the likelihood of their moving from the lowest fifth of income to the top quintile, Americans were optimistic; those in the other countries were mostly pessimistic. People living in the southeast of the United States were the most optimistic, despite being the part of the country with some of the highest poverty rates. People who get welfare from the government there are seen by many—including by many poor—as in front of them in life's line. Americans continue to show a strong belief in hard work producing upward mobility, our so-called meritocracy(19).

Even if you are not poor, you are still afflicted with worse health for living in the United States. This point, raised in Chapter 1, is the most difficult concept for people to accept. We are brought up in the United States with an individualist mentality, believing if we try hard enough anyone can accomplish almost anything. By that logic, the concept that by living in the United States your health is compromised makes no sense. If you are White, well educated with many degrees from prestigious institutions, have a substantial income, see your doctor regularly, and practice all the good health behaviors, you must be exempt from the ideas presented in this book, right? Wrong. An individual who meets these criteria will be healthier than the poorer, the less educated, and people of color, but not as healthy as comparable people in many other nations. Consider the quote from page 3 of the IOM's 2013 monograph(20) mentioned in Chapter 1: "Americans with healthy behaviors or those who are white, insured, college-educated, or in upper-income groups appear to be in worse health than similar groups in comparison countries." We should have among our residents some of the healthiest and longest lived people in the world. Our high levels of poverty, as well as inequality, however, are major factors responsible for not having the healthiest and oldest living here.

A comprehensive 2021 study, by Schwandt and colleagues, considered mortality rates by poverty status for U.S. Blacks and Whites as well as people in six European nations: England, France, Germany, Netherlands, Norway and Spain, grouped together (20). Figure 4.1 shows working age (20-64 years) mortality for the year 2018, comparing income-poverty rates in areas each having approximately 5% of the population. U.S. Whites generally had lower adult mortality than U.S. Blacks, with the poorest third of Blacks having higher death rates than any of the White groups. All six European countries had lower mortality at every level of poverty ranking. The grey lines at the bottom represent each of the individual six countries and the solid black line their average Note the less steep slope of that average line, showing the socioeconomic gradient between mortality and income is less steep than either of

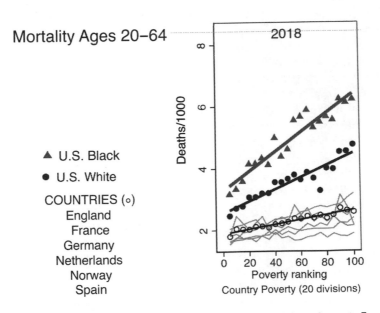

Figure 4.1 Mortality, 2018, ages 20–64, U.S. Blacks, Whites and those from six European countries(21).

the heavier U.S. Black or White lines. The effect of poverty on death rates was substantial for both U.S. racialized groups, in sharp contrast with rates for the Europe nations. Poverty impacts European mortality much less than in the U.S. largely because of significant safety nets there. Racism's impacts will be considered in greater detail in Chapter 6. Notice how at the lowest poverty ranking in 2018, U.S. Whites do not approach the average mortality in the six European nations. Both poverty and inequality kill too many Americans. This figure represents the outcomes of just one study showing that the health of all of us living in the United States is impacted by the inequality with which we live.

Another study looked at the health outcomes of privileged Americans, those living in the highest-income counties, and compared their health outcomes with all residents in 12 other rich nations: Australia, Austria, Canada, Denmark, Finland, France, Germany, Japan, the Netherlands, Norway, Sweden, and Switzerland(22). Whites in the top 1% income brackets still had worse infant and maternal mortality as well as lower survival from colon or breast cancer, leukemia, or heart attacks. Again, our cherry-picked healthiest don't compare with average folk in other nations. Affluent Americans can't escape an early death. There are many other studies supporting these ideas.

Poverty and Moral Decay

Moral decay in the United States limits our ability to address poverty. Consider an experience in Nepal that brought home this lesson.

In 1978, I was crossing a high Himalayan pass (Thorung La at 17,500 feet) to get from one valley to the next on a newly opened route to update my trekking guidebook. At the last hut at 14,000 feet where trekkers slept, I heard that the body of a Nepali porter lay frozen near the pass. The next morning, I came across the scantily clad corpse lying in the snow. This person had worked as a porter for a trekking group that was making the trip from Manang over the pass to the Kali Gandaki Valley. He was a lowlander peasant who was eager to earn some money. He got the job but had little clothing to protect himself from the severe elements in the mountains. A storm came in, and the Nepali head of the workers said they had to rush over the snowy pass so they would not be stranded. He hoped others would provide clothing for those who didn't have enough. Instead, everyone tended to their own needs and the ill-fated Nepali froze to death.

A 1983 *Harvard Business Review* article titled, "The Parable of the Sadhu," told the story of another's similar experience(23). A scantily clad pilgrim or *sadhu* (holy man) was making his way up the same pass. The author—a managing director of Morgan Stanley, the Wall Street giant, and ordained elder of the United Presbyterian Church—came across this holy man during his ascent. He passed him and hoped that others below him would help him not freeze to death. The author said he was too concerned about his own stamina and avoiding altitude sickness to stop and assist. He later reflected on the moral dilemma this decision raised, and the individual versus the group ethic. He wrote about how corporations follow the goals of their executives and shareholders and have no interest in the plight of others who might be affected by these goals. What if his companion and he had carried the *sadhu* down to safety and made sure he was taken care of? He reasoned that both he and his companion were physically stressed and just wanted to cross the pass. He hoped someone else would take the responsibility. Corporations look out only for their bottom line (or profit margin) rather than being morally responsible. In the United States today, there is no one to take care of the poor and marginalized, except for a small number of charitable organizations and a few government programs. The government has mostly disowned responsibility for all but the richest of its citizens. COVID-19 has provided temporary assistance to some, but many more benefits for the richest.

Conclusions

Having poverty in a society leads to worse health for everyone, not just those impoverished but also the well-off. Recognizing such concepts requires looking at complex mortality data. This conflicts with beliefs characteristic of an individualist meritocracy culture that values hard work and personal initiative. America has more poverty than other rich nations and thus worse health.

We will learn more about poverty being bad for your health in subsequent chapters. Being poor in early life is the worst tragedy that can befall us.

Questions to Consider and Discuss

1. Given the huge role of poverty in determining health outcomes, how might we enshrine poverty as a critical disability in the Americans With Disability Act?
2. Does poverty represent a moral failing of a society, or something resulting from individual actions or the lack thereof?

Notes

1. Caste is something you are born into and cannot change. Class reflects a status ascribed by society and is theoretically subject to change in one's lifetime and across generations.
2. And now, this point would be expanded to include access to the internet, something the COVID pandemic brought to public awareness as children required computers and internet connections in order to be schooled and adults required the internet to earn a living.

3. There are certain cancers, such as malignant melanoma, for which this isn't true. This cancer is more common amongst those who get more sun exposure, so-called "sun birds," who tend to be wealthy and seek sunny vacation sites.

References

1. Foege WH. The Fears of the Rich, the Needs of the Poor: My Years at the CDC. Baltimore: Johns Hopkins University Press; 2018.
2. Marmot M. Status Syndrome - How Our Position on the Social Gradient Affects Longevity and Health. London: Bloomsbury; 2004.
3. Sapolsky RM. Why Zebras Don't Get Ulcers: The Acclaimed Guide to Stress, Stress-Related Diseases and Coping. 3rd edition. New York, NY: Henry Holt; 2004.
4. Sahlins M. Stone Age Economics. New York, NY: Aldine; 1972.
5. Scott JC. Against the Grain: a Deep History of the Earliest States. New Haven: Yale University Press; 2017.
6. Suzman J. Affluence Without Abundance. New York, NY: Bloomsbury; 2017.
7. Graeber D, Wengrow D. The Dawn of Everything: a New History of Humanity. New York, NY: Farrar, Straus and Giroux; 2021.
8. Cohen MN. Health and the Rise of Civilization. New Haven: Yale University Press; 1989.
9. Wisman, JD. The Origins and Dynamics of Inequality: Sex, Politics, and Ideology. New York, NY, Oxford University Press; 2022.
10. Larsen CS. Biological Changes in Human Populations With Agriculture. Annual Review of Anthropology. 1995;24:185–213.
11. Cohen MN. The Emergence of Health and Social Inequalities in the Archaeological Record. In: Strickland SS, Shetty PS, editors. Human Biology and Social Inequality: 39th Symposium Volume of the Society for the Study of Human Biology. Cambridge: Cambridge University Press; 1998. pp. 249–71.
12. Ringen S. Poverty in the Welfare State? In: Erikson R, editor. The Scandinavian Model: Welfare States and Welfare Research. Armonk, N.Y.: M.E. Sharpe; 1987. pp. 122–38.
13. Joyce R, Ziliak JP. Relative Poverty in Great Britain and the United States, 1979–2017. Fiscal Studies. 2019;40(4):485–518.
14. UNICEF Innocenti Research Centre. *Innocenti Report Card* No.1, June 2000.'A league table of child poverty in rich nations'. Florence: UNICEF; 2000.
15. Phipps S. Values, Policies and the Well-Being of Young Children: a Comparison of Canada, Norway and the United States. In: Vleminckx K, Smeeding TM, editors. Child Well-Being, Child Poverty and Child Policy in Modern Nations: What Do We Know? Bristol: Policy Press; 2001. pp. 79–98.
16. Pew Center on the States. One in 100: Behind Bars in America 2008. Washington, DC: Pew Charitable Trusts; 2008.
17. Heidary F, Rahimi A, Gharebaghi R. Poverty as a Risk Factor in Human Cancers. Iranian Journal of Public Health. 2013;42(3):341–3.
18. Alesina A, Stantcheva S, Teso E. Intergenerational Mobility and Preferences for Redistribution. American Economic Review. 2018;108(2):521–54.
19. Markovits D. The Meritocracy Trap: How America's Foundational Myth Feeds Inequality, Dismantles the Middle Class, and Devours the Elite. New York, NY: Penguin Press; 2019.

20. Woolf SH, Aron L, editors. U.S. Health in International Perspective: Shorter Lives, Poorer Health: The National Academies Press; 2013.

21. Schwandt H, Currie J, Bär M, Banks J, Bertoli P, Bütikofer A, et al. Inequality in Mortality between Black and White Americans by Age, Place, and Cause and in Comparison to Europe, 1990 to 2018. Proceedings of the National Academy of Sciences. 2021;118(40): e2104684118.

22. Emanuel, EJ, Gudbranson, E, Van Parys, J, Gørtz, M, Helgeland, J, Skinner J. Comparing Health Outcomes of Privileged US Citizens with Those of Average Residents of Other Developed Countries. JAMA Internal Medicine. 2021;181(3):339–44.

23. McCoy BH. The Parable of the Sadhu. Harvard Business Review. 1983;61(5):103–8.

Chapter 5

Early Life Lasts a Lifetime

In my beginning is my end.

T.S. Eliot, Four Quartets

As we go from the erection to the resurrection, how we are ushered into life determines how we leave it. Our early lives as individuals affect our entire lifetimes' health—one of two key ideas in this book, along with the adverse impact of economic inequality. We learned early on in the pandemic that certain groups of people, primarily those with poor health from conception to age two, were more likely to suffer serious health consequences from the SARS-CoV-2 infection. The effect was produced because they were more likely to become infected than others and, if infected, to have more serious symptoms. The search to understand the most basic origins of our health, good or bad, is every bit as important as the quest to understand all we can about the COVID-19 pandemic.

When Our Individual Health Begins

In the early 1970s, I was at Stanford University Medical School. Stanford was a leading center for treating heart disease—manifested as heart attacks and heart failure—with the biggest and best heart transplant program in the world. Doctors developing these heroic measures saved countless lives, but they did not ask the upstream questions about why heart disease had become so common.

Pursuing my studies in medicine, I came across research conducted in the 1950s of postmortem exams on U.S. soldiers who died in the Korean War. Many of these men were in their 20s when their autopsies were performed. A significant number demonstrated atherosclerosis, a narrowing of the coronary arteries feeding the heart muscle and associated with later heart attacks(1). The vessels clog up, and the heart muscle dies. The thinking at Stanford and elsewhere in the early 1970s was that heart attacks resulted from eating too much fat, smoking cigarettes, and not getting enough exercise. Yet young soldiers should not have developed diseased coronary

DOI: 10.4324/9781003315889-6

arteries, as they hadn't been exposed to enough unhealthy behaviors over a long enough period for these physical effects to occur. Combat causalities during the Vietnam War showed similar findings(2). The studies suggested that atherosclerosis begins in childhood and progresses with age. But why?

The concept that chronic diseases such as heart disease, kidney disease, diabetes, and other such conditions have their origins in early life didn't grab me for another 25 years. "If they can get you asking the wrong questions," Thomas Pynchon wrote in *Gravity's Rainbow*, "they don't have to worry about answers." Our understanding of life depends on the questions we ask. The mainstream belief was—and still is—that chronic diseases come about as a result of adult risk factors. This thinking began in the 1940s in Framingham, Massachusetts, prompted by the rising rates of U.S. heart disease. The Framingham study, which is still ongoing and in its third generation of researching participants, originally enrolled two-thirds of the town's citizens aged 29 to 62 who were followed throughout their lives to see who developed coronary artery disease. They found that men with high blood pressure, obesity, high cholesterol, and smoking habits were at greatest risk(3).

The researchers coined the term "risk factors for heart disease." These studies led to a large industry devoted to reducing those risk factors in the adult population. This wasn't necessarily the wrong approach; controlling high blood pressure, decreasing cholesterol, and eliminating smoking can lower deaths from heart disease. Getting people to stop behavior associated with disease progression has long been a predominant perspective of health promotion.

Consider societal influence on health behavior related to smoking habits in the United States. When cigarette smoking was banned in places such as restaurants and workplaces in the 1980s, marked declines in smoking occurred. Deaths from heart disease have similarly been reduced, dropping 68% from the rate in 1958 to that in 2010. It was an important but limited success: Although smoking rates have been reduced, today nicotine addiction is seen primarily in the poorer echelons of American society, who already suffer poorer health.

The goal of modifying the personal behaviors targeted by the risk factor approach impacted how I approached my own patients for several decades. I believed that people's health was almost entirely dictated by their choices, behaviors, and medical care. I considered cigarette smoking the most egregious habit anyone could have. Diet and exercise were also of paramount importance, and I urged my patients to eat better and move more. I was a vegetarian, exercised regularly, and prided myself on my low cholesterol level. If I could do it, so could others.

My views were reinforced by my experiences at work. Many patients I saw in the emergency department were there for smoking-related diseases, including heart attacks and chronic lung disease. Some smokers consumed five to six packs of cigarettes a day. One six-pack-a-day smoker I encountered would get up every hour at night to smoke a cigarette or two.

I tried various methods of advising smokers to quit their cigarette habits over the years, usually to no avail. Frustrated one day, I suggested to a patient that instead of cutting back, he should smoke more, as it would give the hospital more business. I was a profound believer in the connection between personal behaviors and health outcomes. How, then, did I come to change that perspective?

Population Health

A more important question than asking how we can influence people to change their bad health habits is to ask why they started them in the first place. In 1994, I was browsing in San Francisco's UCSF medical bookstore and came across a book of essays entitled, *Why Are Some People Healthy and Others Not? The Determinants of Health of Populations*(4). The title itself asked a critical question. More than 30 years after the individual risk factor approach was adopted, the book's authors suggested that health is more strongly influenced by the population in which one lives than by individual risk factors. The theoretical approach the authors took was termed, "population health." Population health looked at trying to improve collective health and represented what the authors described as "a paradigm shift in the scholarship of health."

This book was my first direct exposure to the socioeconomic gradient in health—poorer people having poorer health, and that the difference in health outcomes between richer and poorer populations has been increasing over the last century. There in Chapter 1, Robert Evans said medical care had not reduced the effect of the socioeconomic gradient. He also discussed how many infectious diseases declined substantially long before the advent of effective treatment with antibiotics and prevention through immunizations. In Chapter 2, I described the article by Kass who pointed out that declines in deaths from infections such as tuberculosis, diphtheria, scarlet fever, whooping cough, and measles occurred long before effective treatments (antibiotics) and preventive measures (immunizations) had become available(5). Kass said this decline resulted from the improvement in socioeconomic circumstances and standards of living, not medical care. He called it "the most important happening in the history of the health of man." Similar U.S. death declines were seen before the immunization was available.

Studies in Minnesota observed deaths from tuberculosis (TB) of the lung over a hundred years. In the early 1900s, Minnesota opened sanatoriums, mostly in the country, where people with TB could be housed, well fed, and cared for in isolated environments that prevented the spread of infection. After this practice was adopted, TB death rates plummeted(6). It wasn't until the late 1940s that effective antibiotic treatments for TB were developed, and by then, most of the declines in deaths had already occurred. Something more important was taking place: Improved living conditions.

As I read *Why Are Some People Healthy and Others Not?* I came to appreciate a broader view of disease. Chapter 1 includes graphs depicting increases in life expectancy between 1960 and 1990 for Japan, France, Germany, Sweden, and the United States. Japan's rapid rise in longevity was clear: By 1978, Japan had the world's longest life expectancy. During the same 30-year period, U.S. life expectancy began to fall behind the other four nations. Evans noted that "Japanese smokers [seemed] less likely to develop lung cancer than their western counterparts." The chapter concludes by questioning the validity of "the simplistic repair shop model of health and health care on which most current health policy is based."

Despite the impact this book had on my thinking, in my medical practice, I remained convinced that the main reason my patients were getting sick was because of the lifestyle choices they were making. Longstanding beliefs are resistant to change. It would take a few decades for the concepts I read to sink in. But reading *Why Are Some People Healthy and Others Not?,* my understanding of the problem had been nudged in a new direction—one that led me to seek out one of the book's contributors, Professor Clyde Hertzman, at the University of British Columbia, to learn what impacted the health trajectory from conception to death.

Dr. Hertzman found that latent factors, those conditions present in early life, continued to strongly influence one's health throughout life. He also considered "pathway events" and "cumulative factors." Pathway events include achieved education level, job category, and socioeconomic status that determined life's trajectories. Cumulative factors comprise the number and duration of bad health behaviors such as injecting drugs and the amount of income earned over many years—where greater income improves health outcomes. Hertzman studied the 1958 British Birth Cohort, a project that followed everyone born in England during that first week of March(7).

Most of the more than 17,000 people born then have not yet died, so proxy measures, self-assessed health, are used instead of mortality. At age 33, the influence of latent factors (between birth and age 7) affects health as much as the pathway and cumulative factors combined. Half of what produces health in adulthood were the latent factors. These include birthweight, height, and social/emotional status as assessed by teachers at age 7, as well as being read to by parents. Early life conditions are strongly linked to adult health. Some of the "medicine" we desperately need in our own country must be administered in this early period, for them to become healthy adults. That is not the prevailing perspective here.

After meeting with Clyde, I considered, "What are the right questions to ask? What factors influence that process?" To find out more, I invited Clyde to a Public Health Grand Rounds at my School of Public Health at the University of Washington in Seattle. The title proposed was, "Another Tale from the Frozen North: Evolution of the Concept of 'Population Health' in Canada and Its Impact on Public Policy." Although "population health" is widely used today, in 1998, the concept was considered vague and confusing and the event's organizers pressed him to change the title of the talk. Hertzman stood firm with his title.

The organizers' concerns proved needless. At the packed Grand Rounds, Professor Hertzman talked about the social foundations of what makes some populations healthier than others. There I first heard the phrase, "Prisoners of the Proximate." This phrase relates back to the Framingham study on adulthood risk factors associated with heart disease and other chronic conditions. In our flawed thinking, we tend to examine and vilify behaviors that are closely linked—proximate—to diseases, such as smoking, diet, drug use, and sedentary lifestyles, but fail to ask why people engage in those behaviors in the first place. Hertzman highlighted how the current vision of our collective responsibility as a society begins when children go to school. But if we are to improve the health of our children and the adults they become, societal responsibility needs to begin at birth, conception, or even earlier.

Professor Hertzman spent the remaining years of his life popularizing the Early Development Instrument (EDI), which works to motivate communities to recognize their collective responsibility for their children's health in early life. He worked tirelessly until his death in 2013, visiting towns throughout British Columbia to make people consider how effectively their communities were engaging with their children's development compared to others, and to inspire them to make improvements. While society has been slow to heed his call, his impact on our scholarly understanding of the social origins of disease was great. And it was through his work, and our continued communications, that my own thinking on the issue went from a nudge in the right direction, to a kick in the pants that would radically change how I not only understood the issues intellectually, but more importantly, how, as a practicing physician, I understood my patients. Their behaviors, I came to see, were mostly not their choice nor could they be changed through willpower alone. Their health-related choices and behaviors were rooted in broader social factors that few understand today.

The term population health has become commonplace, and early life conditions are recognized by many experts as vital for a society's health. The life course approach addresses this critical period acknowledging that cumulative exposures resulting from various bad health behaviors in adulthood influence health outcomes as well. Healthy or unhealthy behavior in adulthood, however, will generally not override early life influences on an individual's health outcomes.

Fetal Origins of Adult Diseases

Hertzman introduced me to the work of Dr. David Barker on the role gestation plays in future health. An upstream thinker, Barker, also wondered why some people were healthy and other's not. In 1986, he noted the association between heart disease mortality rates in England and Wales and infant mortality rates present 45 years earlier, which he took as evidence of early life influences on heart disease. He argued that poor nutrition during pregnancy—leading to low birthweight—was an important factor in later development of heart disease. Barker found birth records of men born between 1911 and 1930 in Hertfordshire, England, that included weight at birth and at one year. He then tracked these people in adulthood and, in 1989, reported that those with the lowest birthweight and weight at one year had the highest rates of death from heart disease(8).

Birthweight measures development in the womb. Barker's findings that low birthweight (less than 5.5 lb. or 2500 g.) and poor growth in the first year of life lead to higher rates of death from heart disease later in life were initially termed the "Barker Hypothesis" by skeptics. Now, his conclusions are recognized by many scientists as part of the fetal origins of adult health paradigm.

Low birthweight is a major risk factor in many other diseases in adulthood. Diseases of the lung (including cancer), kidney, diabetes, high blood pressure, obesity, decreased immunity to infections, and many others that plague us as we age have their origins in early life. Brain development is compromised. Mental health is impaired, with an increased risk of depression and anxiety. Poorer people and those compromised by racism have higher rates of low birthweight, further amplifying the relationship.

Such early life conditions impact how COVID affects us. One Spanish study looking at SARS-CoV-2 infections concludes, "Our data suggest that low birthweight increases the risk of severe COVID-19 in non-elderly adults. This new information further supports the importance of early life events in adult diseases."(9) Low birthweight by itself may lead to obesity, high blood pressure, and other conditions which impact the seriousness of COVID. Younger people born with low birthweight have compromised immunity and an increased susceptibility to SARS-CoV-2 infection and more serious COVID-19. Many of the dangers posed by the infection stem from low birthweight that compromises organ development, including the lungs, heart and kidneys.

SARS-CoV-2 infection during pregnancy can also result in preterm deliveries and low birthweight as well as increases in maternal mortality, leading to generational impairments(10). Fetuses and those very young during the pandemic may have compromised health as they age(11). This effect has been documented for the 1918 flu(12, 13). In the United States, being a fetus in the second trimester of gestation (middle of pregnancy) of the influenza pandemic peak resulted in more heart disease in adulthood, and more diabetes if in the third trimester. More depression also resulted from this exposure, and men did not grow as tall. Various studies in other countries support the concept that being young during that pandemic compromised the health that could be achieved in later life. We can expect compromised health for those who were fetuses, infants, and young children during the COVID-19 pandemic, as they age.

We've already discussed Japan's rapid rise in health and status as the longest-lived nation on Earth. Yet surprisingly, Japan has a high rate of low birthweight infants. How can this fact be reconciled with the fetal origins theory?

I posed the paradox of Japan to Barker. He said Japanese babies with low birthweights tend to be proportionate rather than having the large head and scrawny body typical of low birthweight babies elsewhere. Being born of low birthweight, especially very low birthweight (<1500 g. or 3.3 lb.), in Japan does appear to compromise adult health. Examples include developing kidney disease at a young age and reduced cognitive ability. But the effects appear to be less than expected. There is something special about the health of the Japanese that doesn't follow the typical guidelines considered important for health. These include their rates of smoking, as well as other issues we will discuss later that break many so-called rules for producing good health. We must consider facts that don't fit the theory to better understand health production.

David Barker speculated that the womb may be even more important than the home environment after birth. This perspective was not something presented in medical school nor in my later schooling—and still is not. Why is the in utero period so important in determining adult health?

No mythical stork delivers newborns to their mothers. We all started off with our father's sperm fertilizing our mother's ovum to produce a zygote. That single cell divides into two, and then, each of those cells divides into two again. The process repeats itself about 42 times, so a newborn emerges with over 4 trillion cells(8).

There are only about 5 further cycles of cell division required to produce you, the adult reader (totaling 140 trillion cells). What happens during growth and development is that some cells have a life span considerably shorter than your own. Blood cells, skin cells, male sperm cells, and intestinal lining cells die off, to be replaced by new cells. The neurons in your brain and nervous system and ova in ovaries are never replaced. Some, such as muscle cells in the heart, are only rarely replaced.

An enormous amount of cell division, organ modeling, and other activity occurs in the first nine months of life. After birth, the rate of cell division slows down. When cells are dividing, they are sensitive to a variety of outside influences. If there isn't sufficient nutrition for developing cells, their division will be compromised. Ionizing radiation can affect cell division, and a whole host of chemicals can influence the process. Some prescription drugs can cause birth defects or cancer in the baby, so their use must be limited during pregnancy. Infections such as rubella can cause birth defects and brain damage if the mother contracts the virus in the first 20 weeks of pregnancy. Zika virus infections during pregnancy can cause brain development issues. The full impact of SARS-CoV-2 on pregnancy is still unclear, although we do know the virus leads to low birthweight and preterm deliveries. Maternal stress may also play a role. Psychosocial stress during pregnancy affecting cell and organ growth is now recognized as producing many negative health effects in the newborn. Maternal anxiety from worrying about the pandemic as well as the added stress of being pregnant during this unprecedented time in modern history will undoubtedly have long-term effects.

Consider: If we want to make a healthy 25-year-old person, would we focus on the first nine months after conception, or on the next 25 years? Or, to put it another way, if we wanted to efficiently inflict *damage* on such a person, would the focus be on the first nine months (with 42 cycles of cell division) or on the next 25 years (with only 5 cycles)? The answer to that question is becoming clearer as more research unfolds: Conditions from conception to birth are extremely important for the health of the adults those infants will become. No one can return to the womb to fix their future health. But there are changes society can make for better health for the unborn by improving maternal and prenatal health.

The effect on fetuses was unintentionally tested during the last mid-century. A natural experiment, the Dutch Hunger Winter, allowed us to gauge how nutritional stress during pregnancy later impacted adult health of the infants who were *in utero* during the period from November 1944 to April 1945 within World War II(14). Then, with the war ravaging Europe, daily rations in Holland for adults fell below 1000 calories. Pregnant women were intended to get extra food, but when a famine gripped the region, this became impossible.

Fetuses who were exposed to the famine during the early months of their gestation, in contrast to those born before the famine, were more likely to have diabetes, mental disorders, and a lipid blood profile (high cholesterol and tri-glycerides), subjecting them to high risk of coronary artery disease, as well as increased stress sensitivity, female obesity, and many other chronic diseases in adulthood. Those exposed in mid-gestation were prone to lung and kidney disease and diabetes. Those exposed in late gestation had higher rates of diabetes. These findings correspond to periods in the uterus when various organs are being formed. What's more, the damage isn't restricted to a single generation—it perpetuates into successive generations.

When those Dutch famine-affected infants became adults and had children of their own, that second generation tended to have health problems in later life, including diabetes and obesity. This demonstrates the intergenerational transmission of health from those affected by the famine in utero to their own children. Recent studies suggest that epigenetic factors, meaning the variation in gene expression that results from various social and physical environmental exposures, influence the health of subsequent generations, a point discussed further in Chapter 7.

The ovum your father's sperm fertilized was made in your mother's ovary. Women are born with all the ova they will ever have, so the ovum that begat you developed in your grandmother's womb. In other words, you started life in your maternal grandmother's womb, where the egg that produced you originated. So your maternal grandmother's circumstances—her health, her living conditions, and her social relations—impact your health much later.

While much of our focus is on population health measured by death rates, a proxy measure is average height in a society. In more egalitarian societies, food is more equally distributed and average height is higher. In the 19th century, Americans were among the tallest in the world. But over the decades, as we have become less egalitarian, we've become shorter. Average height in the United States now lags behind that in most longer lived nations. As with other measures of health, a woman's height is related to her own mother's height and to her birthweight, as well as genetic factors. Intergenerational transmission occurs: The grandmother's height helps determine the mother's height, which in turn affects the infant's birthweight(15).

Maternal health is important. Yet surprisingly, many studies show that prenatal care has limited impact on that birth's outcome(16). While society must provide such care to all pregnant women, especially now that we have the technology to treat and even reverse some health problems of both mother and fetus, important outcomes of pregnancy have already been determined by conditions the mother has faced since her own beginnings.

The challenge in the Dutch Hunger Winter was primarily nutritional stress, but many other kinds of stress are common in modern life and affect health. Natural experiments examining the impact of the attacks on the World Trade Center towers on September 11, 2001, or of Hurricane Katrina in 2005, provide insights on the effect of psychological stress. Births to women who were pregnant on 911, both those living in New York City and women living far from the destruction, show more low birthweight and preterm deliveries(17). Social stress from harassment or racism has also impacted birthweight and premature delivery. The results of the U.S. presidential election in 2016, arguably one of the most stressful election in decades and one in which people of color were routinely targeted for harassment and abuse, produced more low birthweight babies born to people of color. A California study looked at police killings between 2005 and 2017, finding that if you were Black and pregnant near a police killing of an unarmed Black, you were more likely to have a low birthweight baby than if you were Black and pregnant but had not been close to such a killing(18). Being in the first trimester and within a mile or two had the greatest risk.

Rates of self-reported stress in the United States are among the highest in the world. By living in this very stressed nation, your chances of delivering a low birthweight baby are high—and one of the most vulnerable organs stress can affect is the human brain.

Brain development is compromised for low birthweight infants, often limiting one's educational achievement that in turn can lead to worse health outcomes. All children born in Florida from 1992 to 2002 who attended public schools had their birthweights tracked as well as how they performed on standardized tests from grades three to eight. Higher test scores corresponded with higher birthweights, up to a peak of 9.5 pounds, with a slight decline above that. There were ranges of outcomes for each birthweight, so if newborns weighed only two pounds, they did not all perform poorly in school, but were just more likely to do so than a higher birthweight baby. These outcomes did not depend on the quality of teaching in the schools. Because there were over 1.3 million children in this study, the results had very high levels of statistical significance(19).

Both birthweights and maternal education were related to test scores. At each level of a mother's education, higher birthweights are related to higher test scores, with the best test scores found in the group of infants whose mothers were college graduates. Next were those mothers with some college, and below them were high school graduates. The lowest test score outcomes were for the children of mothers who did not complete high school. Again, for each mother's educational group, being of low birthweight does not doom the child to a low test score; it is just more likely(20). The point is not that individuals might not fare well if they were born with low birthweight. As a group, those born with low birthweight are more likely to be disadvantaged in terms of physical and mental health, as well as cognitive skills. My mother only had four years of schooling, yet I did well in tests. There are similar ethnic divides with Black mothers faring worse than White.

A mother's education level is a measure of her socioeconomic status. The relationship between birthweight and later test scores illustrates the socioeconomic gradient: Poorer mothers are more likely to have low birthweight babies who themselves, when they grow up, are also likely to be poor and have low birthweight babies. It is a challenging cycle to break.

Parental investment in a low birthweight baby can make considerable differences in that child's outcomes. But investment by considerably less educated parents, or poorer parents, does not show the same benefits obtainable by more educated parents. Some of this has to do with poverty issues and schools that we discussed in the previous chapter as well as preschools. COVID impacts low birthweight and will affect subsequent educational outcomes as future research is almost certain to demonstrate.

Although birth outcomes are not destiny, we are not all born equal. What happens in the next few years of life impacts adult life as well.

Early Life after Birth

The United Nations Children's Agency, UNICEF, tracks child outcomes in rich countries. They present league tables, which are comparisons of various outcomes among rich nations. Child well-being measures include child poverty, child injury, child abuse or maltreatment, deaths, homicide, teenage births, educational disadvantage, obesity, and other summary measures such as family and peer relationships. In most measures, the United States is either the worst or second worst among the 27 countries listed(21). We can do better.

The practice of raising children used to be passed on without question from one generation to the next. Parents mirrored behaviors they were exposed to as children, and grandparents—especially grandmothers—helped as well. Below we will see how the U.S. economy has changed, so with both parents working, parenting becomes more difficult.

Child upbringing styles around the world vary tremendously. But one universal feature found in all is that a failure to nurture children at an early age produces adults who fail to function well in society.

A natural experiment points out what happens with zero parenting. In the 1970s, Romanian leader Nicolae Ceauşescu began policies to increase fertility, with the goal of producing more people to promote economic growth. Abortion was banned; women had to produce children. Communal living in urban apartment complexes became the norm, focusing on the worker rather than the family. Newborns, infants, and children were abandoned. As orphanages were set up to house these unwanted children, horrific policies ensued. Infants and toddlers were left unattended in cribs and sometimes even chained to them, as a result of the incredibly imbalanced ratio of children to staff members available to care for them(22).

After Ceauşescu's execution in 1989, outside news sources revealed that hundreds of thousands of children suffered in very poorly run state institutions. International humanitarian attempts were made to improve conditions for these unfortunate children, but the damage was already done. Despite subsequent improved living conditions, the situation left many children with profound deficits, including serious mental and physical disorders. Even after being adopted by nurturing parents, health issues persisted. Early parenting matters.

The socioeconomic status of the parents, both when the child is still in the womb and for the first few years afterward, matters for that child's adult health. The richer or more educated the parents, the better the adult health outcomes for the child(23). Life's chances are rigged: a better start predicts a better outcome. Some people with unhealthy starts do well later in life, but these are the exceptions.

Our 1958 British Birth Cohort study found that around half of adult health is determined in the first seven years. The first thousand days after conception is now seen as the most critical period(24). As we will see below, societies that privilege the period up to a child's second birthday will have healthier children than those who delay interventions until after the child reaches school. To maximize brain development and produce healthy children then focus on the first thousand days. Understanding something about human prehistory clarifies why these thousand days are so critical to our development.

Recall the long paleolithic era. Diets were relatively high in protein and low in carbohydrates with variation depending on where people lived: Paleo-Eskimos consumed almost exclusive animal intakes, while Bushmen ate more plant carbohydrates. As humans traveled north, leaving Africa and settling in more northern regions, they took up pastoralism and agriculture. With the development of animal husbandry and agriculture, diets changed to include more, mostly unrefined, carbohydrates. Obesity, previously absent, began to appear, but was initially limited to richer populations and individuals who didn't have to labor to produce their food. Today, with modern technologies that further reduce our physical labor and how we obtain and store our food, societies have undergone a nutrition transition, with relatively cheap, calorie dense, refined carbohydrate foods constituting our main source of nutrition(25). We now have higher calorie consumption and resulting obesity throughout the globe, but especially in the United States where fast food and processed ingredients are popular. Unsurprisingly, the United States is the most obese nation today.

The fetus lives in a womb with a view; namely, signals of the external environment are picked up by the mother and transferred to the fetus(13). Metabolic syndrome, a cluster of findings that lead to heart disease and diabetes, starts when the fetus gets stress signals from the mother that a difficult world awaits outside. Born often prematurely with a low birthweight, the baby engages in catch-up growth that leads to today's chronic diseases. Food has become a stress reliever, and modern society is increasingly stressful, so we continue to overeat.

John Bowlby, a British psychiatrist who studied orphans after the Second World War, found that the presence of a single supportive caregiver (including what he called a mother substitute) who responded to the infant's needs was needed for what he termed "secure attachment." Secure attachment allows children to self-regulate and be comfortable around strangers(26). If presented with many different caregivers, the infant was more likely to be uncomfortable among strangers and exhibit insecure attachment. After the first year, research suggested that a second caregiver supports the attachment process. Ideally, these same caregivers should be present in later years.

Attachment-focused parenting is an option for many today. Such practices include prolonged breastfeeding, co-sleeping, and encouraging the baby to freely explore his or her environment. A competing reality is the practice of outsourcing parenting to enable women an uninterrupted focus on their careers. In either case, what is required is appropriate personal attention directed to the infant and young child.

Yet, parenting requires time. Almost all contemporary nations give new parents time to nurture newborns through paid parental leave(27). Parents are given a set amount of paid time off work to focus on the work of parenting. Only two countries in the world with populations over a million do not provide this benefit. One is the United States, and the other is Papua New Guinea. Sweden gives parents 444 days of leave at full pay after the birth of a baby. The father is *required* to take 13 weeks. More leave can be taken at a lower rate of pay. Day care there, up to 15 hours per week, is free. In Canada, new parents are given a choice between 61 weeks at 33% pay or 35 weeks at 55% pay, which can be stretched out over 18 months. Employers often offer additional pay.

These nations make this investment in their citizens because they understand that paid parental leave improves the health outcomes of future generations.

A study of career mothers by Caitlyn Collins, a sociologist at Washington University, interviewed working mothers in Sweden, Germany, Italy, and the United States(28). The least work–family conflict was seen among the mothers in Sweden, which had generous policy supports for both mothering and their careers. In former East Germany, there was a little more conflict between the demands of work and family, and more still in former West Germany. Italy had similar conflicts as well. These nations all have significant paid parental leave and childcare policies. Collins's study found that without federal paid leave women in the United States had the most problems in working outside the home. They had plenty of stress tying to be perfect moms and, even if working, remained responsible for most of the cooking and upkeep of the home. The European mothers expected and enjoyed considerable help from the government, while the U.S. mothers had no expectation of any kind of state support. American mothers have to do it all by themselves, a demonstration of our individualist mentality.

A few U.S. states now have paid leave policies, although none are as substantial as in most other developed nations. In 2002, California became the first state to enact a paid family leave law. The law led to increased exclusive breastfeeding, with its benefits on health and immunity, mothers spending more time on childcare and fewer infant hospitalizations. Others now include Connecticut, Massachusetts, New Jersey, New York, Rhode Island, and Washington. The national 1993 Family Medical Leave Act grants four months of conditional *unpaid* leave. That's a step in the right direction, but doesn't go very far, as few families can afford to take unpaid leave.

The strongest parents in the United States tend to be those in upper income categories, particularly those who are married, in their 30s, and have college degrees. More prosperous parents can spend more time with their children than can less affluent parents. They spend more time talking with their children and provide stimulating environments. Children of white-collar parents hear three to four times the number of words per hour than children in working-class families(29). The child's exposure to types of words differs based on socioeconomic class. In low-income families, children are more likely to hear cease-and-desist commands: Shut up, don't do that, go away! More educated families tend to listen to the child more attentively and may explain the reasons behind the behavior they're trying to influence. A parent may say, "We don't throw baseballs inside the house because they might break a window," rather than just demand the child not do so or face punishment for disobedience. Engaging word stimulation enhances brain development.

Children from poorer families also tend to perform more poorly in school than children from richer families. We have seen the impact of birthweight and mother's education on poor school performance. The educational performance gap between poorer and richer children in the United States has increased in tandem with the rising rich–poor divide. As discussed in the previous chapter, poor American neighborhoods must spend less money on their schools. They have higher teacher turnover, less skilled teachers, dilapidated schools, overcrowded classrooms, and fewer courses—if any—in science and technology, the arts, and extracurricular programs. We have more poverty than other rich countries, so our schools reflect this inequality. They can't provide the supportive instruction present in other countries where there is a more equitable system for funding schools. COVID has exposed the consequences of our poor schools. As classroom instruction became virtual, many students had limited internet access, as well as a lack of supervision in many homes because both parents continued to work, while wealthier families often hired tutors, or one or both parents had more free time to supervise their children's instruction.

Wealth alone doesn't guarantee optimal development, however. Children in the United States—both rich and poor—are falling behind in academic performance. International comparisons of mathematics, science, and reading competence in the teenage years demonstrate that U.S. children increasingly underperform children in other rich nations. The decline occurs despite school accountability programs which seek to improve school performance and education accessibility. Our compromised beginnings limit what schooling can accomplish.

The United States has the highest rates of single and teen parenthood among rich nations and also has the most single-parent poverty. Teenage girls who drop out of high school in more unequal U.S. states are more likely to be mothers than more highly educated ones. Poorer women are more likely to have low birthweight babies with compromised brain development, who then perform poorly in school. Single parenthood and teen parenthood carry higher risks of poor health for the offspring. Even in Sweden, a country with healthcare for all and very low poverty rates, children in single-parent homes have higher mortality rates than those where there are two parents, and single parents there also have worse health.

Single-parent households are more likely to be poor, and if you were raised in poverty, you are also more likely to develop hypertension as an adult. African American households are disproportionately headed by a single woman. Black men have particularly high blood pressure. Black men in Washington, D.C. who lived with two parents between the ages of 1 and 12 tended to have considerably lower blood pressures as adults than those in single-parent households(30). Both parents can produce a more nurturing environment to facilitate healthy human development, with health advantages in later life.

What impacts of COVID-19 can we expect on young children's developmental, behavioral, and emotional health? The home situation where parents work remotely adds to the stress of child care. Playing with other children has been disrupted, so the socialization expected to occur may not progress smoothly. School instruction has been vastly modified with only speculative effects.

We can expect that children in higher socioeconomic situations will do better than those in more marginalized communities. There will be substantial cross-country variations.

The African proverb "it takes a village to raise a child" reflects the fact that many societies do not expect mothers or parents to rear children alone. The way a society cares for and protects its children defines its moral and social fabric. The United States lacks national support for child rearing, while Scandinavian countries spend up to sixty times as much per capita on childcare than the United States does. With little national support, lower-income American families are less stable, as families move, schools and neighborhoods change, and divorce rates rise. Many children here are exposed to the merry-go-round of three or more maternal figures, a higher number than any other rich nation. American children living in such complex unstable families have more biological stress and worse health. Do parents matter? What kind of parenting is best? One thing we do know is that family instability arising from transitions in family structure and chaos in the home results in worse adult health outcomes than more stable single-parent households.

We began this chapter by challenging the concept that risk factors, certain behaviors or conditions in adulthood, are responsible for chronic diseases, the so-called diseases of aging. These behaviors pale in comparison to more upstream factors, the conditions in early life that impact health in adulthood. But what happens when a child is subjected to something far more extreme than imperfect behaviors? What happens when the behavior a child is subjected to is abuse?

Adverse Childhood Experiences

DeMause began his 1974 book *The History of Childhood* with, "The history of childhood is a nightmare from which we have only recently begun to awaken. The further back in history one goes the lower the level of child care, and the more likely children are to be killed abandoned, beaten, terrorized and sexually abused." Child abuse is the major hidden epidemic of our time(31). Our most common individual health issues today may represent unconscious attempts at dealing with trauma dating back to our earliest years.

The first attempt to systematically explore early life abuse began in the 1970s through a weight reduction program at the Kaiser Permanente San Diego Clinic. Dr. Vincent Felitti treated morbidly obese women with a supervised fasting program which enabled many of these patients to lose a hundred pounds or more in a year. Felitti couldn't understand why so many of them quickly regained their lost weight and dropped out of the program. His discussions with these women revealed that after losing weight, they suddenly became attractive to men. Many had been sexually abused as children, and becoming obese was their way of treating early life trauma by making themselves undesirable to their abusers. Obesity was their body armor. Intrigued by this revelation, Felitti and Dr. Robert Anda developed an Adverse Childhood Experiences (ACEs) study to discover how often these experiences happened and their impacts on adult health.

There were three main categories of ACEs: *abuse* (1) psychological, (2) physical, and (3) sexual; *neglect* (4) emotional and (5) physical; and *household dysfunction* (6) alcoholism or drug use at home, (7) divorce or loss of a biological parent before the age of 18, (8) depression or mental illness in the home, (9) violent treatment of the mother, or (10) an imprisoned household member. The ACE score was the sum of these ten categories of early life experiences.

Two-thirds of the Kaiser population studied had one or more ACEs. The higher the ACE score, the more likely the adult would exhibit alcoholism, injection drug use, mental illness, suicide attempts, memory impairment, teen parenthood, excessive numbers of sexual partners, and serious job problems. A higher ACE score led to an increased rate of early death. Six or more ACEs resulted in a twenty-year shorter life. Higher rates of cancer, obesity, and mental illness in later life occurred among those abused as children.

These findings, published in 1998, with follow-up in 2009, challenged the effect of medical care. Felitti and Anda later discussed their findings in the 2014 book *Chadwick's Child Maltreatment*(32). They say, "Clearly, much of what we see in adult medical practice and as current major public health problems has its origins in what was present but unrecognized in pediatrics. There is a need to move from our current symptom-responsive approach in primary care to the comprehensive approach that was conceived but not attained—what George Engel described as a biopsychosocial approach.[1]" Many factors must be accounted for to understand what conditions an individual has, and what benefits or harms arise from them. We need to address the causes.

ACEs in the Kaiser San Diego population were more prevalent in women than in men. ACEs are more common in poorer families, though they exist across the entire socioeconomic spectrum. More are seen in the southeastern United States where health outcomes are already worse.

ACEs exist around the world. Like many non-mortality measures related to health, they are difficult to characterize and study. Trauma is another term used. ACE reporting is increasing, either a true increase or the result of heightened awareness. What should be the response?

"Gradually, we came to see that asking, listening, and enabling a patient to go home feeling still accepted, is in itself a major intervention," Felitti and Anda wrote. "The clinical practice of asking, listening, and accepting is *doing*."

Questions of how ACEs can be prevented, or the consequences treated, are unresolved. Mainstream media avoid their discussion. Recent U.S. revelations of sexual harassment and abuse on a wide scale make clear that such abuses are mostly perpetrated by men, especially men with considerable power. The #MeToo movement has brought some of these concerns to light so that we might address them. But there is no systemic exploration of child abuse; our youngest remain voiceless.

Dr. Nadine Burke Harris, a San Francisco pediatrician, wrote *The Deepest Well: Healing the Long-Term Effects of Childhood Adversity* where she presents her experiences and efforts(33). Despite no cure for childhood trauma, one can help mitigate its effects. Wider exposure of ACEs' impact is a first step to help victims of child abuse.

What impact has COVID-19 had on ACEs? The relationship of ACEs with COVID-19 Post-Traumatic Stress symptoms (CPTSS—it is too soon to call it a disorder) has been studied among adolescents in rural China and shows the expected relationship with more ACEs producing more CPTSS. Scars from the past make one vulnerable to severe stresses during the pandemic.

Isolation and absence from school along with rising intimate partner violence, a rise in opioid consumption, and the devastating economic impacts portend a rise in ACEs. News reports suggest domestic violence worldwide has increased with the pandemic. As such, we can expect ACEs to rise with the crisis.

Building Strong Children to Prevent Repairing Broken Adults

Frederick Douglass was an African American statesman who, having escaped from slavery, became a leader of the abolitionist movement and campaigned throughout his life for equality of all people regardless of background. In 1855, he had a series of dialogues with White slave owners who could not comprehend that slavery was morally wrong. Following these discussions, he wrote, "It is easier to build strong children than to repair broken men."

Today, we have a huge industry—roughly one-sixth of the total U.S. economy—attending to broken men and women in the repair shop—the medical care business. My work as an emergency doctor for 30 years depended on having damaged people to fix. It is easier to build strong children, and doing so costs a great deal less and ultimately benefits all of society. James Heckman, a Nobel Prize-winning economist, demonstrated the profound returns to investment in early life(34). Social programs which target the earliest years (before age three) have a much greater return on investment than those addressing school, job training, and mending broken adults.

Yet, the United States spends significantly more on middle and late childhood than it does on the early years. Sweden spends more during the first year of life than on any subsequent year and has much better health outcomes than the United States. With COVID, we now have a health crisis in the United States that gives us an opportunity to change our bad outcomes by focusing on children's early years. What kinds of programs or investments are required?

One approach comes from the Perry Preschool Project in Ypsilanti, Michigan. The program investigated high-quality interventions for low-income children. Children aged 3–5 received a 3-hour daily program designed to engage their imagination on mathematics, literacy, and various forms of play, and by providing home-based parenting guidance. These children were compared with a group not in the program. Fifty years later, the children in the program were more likely to do well in school, graduate, get a job, and start a family, than the group without the intervention. Each dollar invested in the program returned 7–8% per year over the lifetime of the child. That payoff of seven to eight dollars for each dollar invested annually is a tremendous rate of return(35).

The U.S. study results were applied in Canada. Quebec, once Canada's poorest province, had exceedingly high social welfare costs and wanted to control them. There was great enthusiasm for the economic benefits promised by the results of the Perry Preschool Project. In 1992, the Quebec government proposed actions over ten years that would set up a culture of preventive actions for the children and families that needed it the most. By 1997, universal day care was offered at $5 per day. Quebec also had 40 weeks of paid maternal leave at 75% of their salary, which can be shared with the father. Health improved. Costs went down. Quebec now has better health outcomes than the healthiest of American states.

The Carolina Abecedarian Project stemmed from the recognition that various forms of adversity in early life, especially social and economic, may permanently affect children through adulthood. It began in North Carolina in 1972 and ran for five years providing infant and toddler care, healthcare, and nutritional support as well as preschool for 111 disadvantaged children. Children in the program were four times more likely to graduate from college than those who weren't. The focus of this project on limiting early life adversity may be the best example of true prevention when it comes to producing better adult health(36).

Nurse–Family Partnerships have nurses in different areas of the United States visiting the homes of low-income mothers having their first child. In one group, nurses began visiting pregnant mothers at home and continued to visit after birth. A comparison group received no visits. Results included an increase in maternal employment and in the father's presence in the household, as well as higher birthweights, over a third fewer injuries to children, and a nearly 50% decrease in child abuse and neglect. Children were two-thirds less likely to have behavioral and intellectual problems by age 6, and there were fewer child arrests by age 15(37). Analogous studies in other countries, including the Netherlands and the United Kingdom, have produced similarly positive results. However, many rich countries offer much more support for early life than available in the United States, so an additional program's impact may be less. Health visitors in the United Kingdom are nurses or midwives who visit all families regularly from pregnancy until the child is two years old. For more vulnerable children, the visits continue to age 5. They are an inbuilt feature of supporting early life there.

A range of other programs demonstrate benefits in reducing low birthweight and improving other early life factors. The U.S. federal WIC, "Women, Infants, and Children," program (also known as Supplemental Nutrition Assistance

Program or SNAP) provides supplemental foods and nutrition education for low-income pregnant women and those caring for infants and children up to the age of five. Our only national program for support of young children has produced positive outcomes such as lower infant mortality especially among African Americans, increased breastfeeding, fewer premature deliveries, and increased birthweight(38).

Reducing the Effects of Child Poverty

Educational levels are closely related to poverty. Considering English-speaking countries such as Canada, Australia, and the United Kingdom reveals that average family incomes for a four-person family among medium and lower educated families are similar in these countries. Highly educated American families, however, have considerably higher incomes than similarly educated families in those nations.

At ages four to five, children in the United States have poorer language and reading skills than in the other three countries(39). Those countries also have a higher proportion of children living with both parents at every level of parental education. We've seen that single parenthood is detrimental to the health of both the child and the parent. These statistics don't imply that it is impossible for some individuals to do well despite their disadvantages—but it's significantly easier to do better in the United Kingdom, Australia, and Canada.

Reading to children and engaging with them, rather than sitting them in front of the television or computer or smartphone, is a part of successful parenting. Fewer parents in the United States read to their children every day than they used to, and primary school children have more screen time. Distractive devices are not effective child-rearing strategies. With more poverty in the United States than in other rich nations, parenting is often outsourced out of necessity, as both parents must work to make ends meet.

The U.S. family environment has changed considerably since the 1970s. Senator Elizabeth Warren, when a Harvard law school professor, examined the economic situation of the average two-parent two-child family in 1970, in which one parent worked in the home, while the other worked outside the home(40). Using data from the Bureau of Labor Statistics' *Consumer Expenditure Survey* Warren looked at their spending, including housing, education, healthcare, and others. She then compared this family to the similar average family in 2000 when both parents worked outside the home. Even with a dual income, the economy had changed so drastically in those three decades that the 2000 family had less money for discretionary expenses such as vacations and non-essential goods, than the 1970 family with only one wage earner!

When looking at the so-called market income, what appears on paychecks, the United States does not have the highest level of poverty. However, after looking at the impact of taxes and transfers, there are considerably more families in poverty in the United States than in the other three nations above. Transfers include government supports such as cash transfers, or welfare payments, and non-cash subsidies for housing and transportation. The government and private agencies provide something of value without requiring the recipient to pay for it. The United States provides considerably fewer transfer payments than the other studied countries. Recent tax cut legislation has resulted in worsening the divide as less advantaged people have higher tax bills relative to their income than their wealthier counterparts. Other rich countries have also provided many more cash benefits during the COVID pandemic than the United States has, suggesting that those hardest hit economically will struggle to regain their economic footing in the post-COVID years.

The End Is in the Beginning

Like a curious three year old asking, "Why?" there is a line of critical reasoning that endlessly asks for the causes of causes. What causes heart disease? Risk factors. What causes risk factors? Early life issues. What causes early life issues? Societal choices. What causes societal choices? And so on. The Public Health Agency of Canada depicts this important chain of reasoning on its website: *What Makes Canadians Healthy or Unhealthy?*(41)

This deceptively simple story speaks to the complex set of factors or conditions that determine the level of health of every Canadian.

Why is Jason in the hospital?
Because he has a bad infection in his leg.

But why does he have an infection?
Because he has a cut on his leg and it got infected.

But why does he have a cut on his leg?
Because he was playing in the junkyard next to his apartment building and there was some sharp, jagged steel there that he fell on.

But why was he playing in a junkyard?
Because his neighborhood is kind of run down. A lot of kids play there and there is no one to supervise them.

But why does he live in that neighborhood?
Because his parents can't afford a nicer place to live.

But why can't his parents afford a nicer place to live?
Because his Dad is unemployed and his Mom is sick.

But why is his Dad unemployed?
Because he doesn't have much education and he can't find a job.

But why ...?
There is nothing comparable on an American federal government website.

Conclusion

Our failing health begins when we don't invest in early childhood. Frederick Douglass's statement holds true today. It is easier to mend our broken children now than it will be to repair the broken adults they become. Nothing produces better outcomes in health and economic security than efforts directed at early life. These interventions prevent or delay the onset of adult diseases, with many other beneficial outcomes.

We must make sure that our children have the support they need to thrive from conception through childhood. For millions of today's youth, that recognition may be too late. But for the well-being of millions more children yet to be born, it will be essential.

A long time ago I learned that every illness has something to teach us. If we don't learn that, then it will keep impacting our lives. COVID provides the lessons we need to prioritize policies impacting early life. What are these lessons, and what are the differences in American health outcomes we must prioritize? We'll explore those questions in the next chapter.

Questions to Consider and Discuss

1. Even among progressives looking broadly at health promotion, the importance of early life is rarely acknowledged. Why might this be?
2. What can be done to gain greater recognition?

Note

1. Engel GL. The need for a new medical model: a challenge for biomedicine. Science. 1977;196(4286):129-36

References

1. Enos WF, Beyer JC. Coronary Artery Disease in Younger Men. JAMA. 1971;218(9): 1434.
2. McNamara JJ, Molot MA, Stremple JF, Cutting RT. Coronary Artery Disease in Combat Casualties in Vietnam. JAMA. 1971;216(7):1185–7.
3. Tsao CW, Vasan RS. The Framingham Heart Study: Past, Present and Future. International Journal of Epidemiology. 2015;44(6):1763–6.
4. Evans RG, Barer ML, Marmor TR, editors. *Why Are Some People Healthy and Others Not?: the Determinants of Health of Populations*. New York, NY: De Gruyter; 1994.
5. Kass EH. Infectious Diseases and Social Change. Journal of Infectious Diseases. 1971; 123(1):110–4.
6. Wilson LG. The Rise and Fall of Tuberculosis in Minnesota: The Role of Infection. Bulletin of the History of Medicine. 1992;66(1):16.
7. Hertzman C, Boyce T. How Experience Gets Under the Skin to Create Gradients in Developmental Health. Annual Review of Public Health. 2010;31(1):329–47.

8. Barker DJP. *Mothers, Babies, and Health in Later Life.* 2nd edition. Edinburgh: Churchill Livingstone; 1998.

9. Crispi F, Crovetto F, Larroya M, Camacho M, Tortajada M, Sibila O, et al. Low Birth Weight as a Potential Risk Factor for Severe COVID-19 in Adults. Scientific Reports. 2021;11(1):2909.

10. Melo GC, Araújo KCGM. COVID-19 Infection in Pregnant Women, Preterm Delivery, Birth Weight, and Vertical Transmission: A Systematic Review and Meta-Analysis. Cadernos De Saúde Pública. 2020;36(7):e00087320.

11. Easterlin MC, Crimmins EM, Finch CE. Will Prenatal Exposure to SARS-CoV-2 Define a Birth Cohort With Accelerated Aging in the Century Ahead? Journal of Developmental Origins of Health and Disease. 2020:1–5.

12. Almond D. Is the 1918 Influenza Pandemic Over? Long-Term Effects of In Utero Influenza Exposure in the Post-1940 U.S. Population. Journal of Political Economy. 2006;114(4):672–712.

13. Paul AM. Origins: How the Nine Months Before Birth Shape the Rest of Our Lives. New York, NY: Free Press; 2010.

14. Roseboom T, de Rooij S, Painter R. The Dutch Famine and Its Long-Term Consequences for Adult Health. Early Human Development. 2006;82(8):485–91.

15. Emanuel I, Kimpo C, Moceri V. The Association of Grandmaternal and Maternal Factors With Maternal Adult Stature. International Journal of Epidemiology. 2004;33(6):1243–8.

16. Kramer MS, Goulet L, Lydon J, Seguin L, McNamara H, Dassa C, et al. Socio-Economic Disparities in Preterm Birth: Causal Pathways and Mechanisms. Paediatric and Perinatal Epidemiology. 2001;15:104–23.

17. Ohlsson A, Shah PS, Knowledge Synthesis Group of Determinants of Preterm/LBW births. Effects of the September 11, 2001 Disaster on Pregnancy Outcomes: a Systematic Review. Acta Obstetricia Et Gynecologica Scandinavica. 2011;90(1):6–18.

18. Legewie J. Police Violence and the Health of Black Infants. Science Advances. 2019; 5:eaax7894.

19. Figlio D, Guryan J, Karbownik K, Roth J. The Effects of Poor Neonatal Health on Children's Cognitive Development. American Economic Review. 2014;104(12): 3921–55.

20. Leonhardt D, Cox A. Heavier Babies Do Better in School New York: New York Times; 2014 [cited 2014 October 10]. Available from: http://www.nytimes.com/2014/10/12/upshot/heavier-babies-do-better-in-school.html.

21. UNICEF Innocenti Research Centre. *Innocenti Report Card 16 Worlds of Influence: Understanding What Shapes Child Well-Being in Rich Countries.* Florence: UNICEF; 2020.

22. Nelson CA, Fox NA, Zeanah CH. Romania's Abandoned Children. Deprivation, Brain Development, and the Struggle for Recovery. Cambridge, Massachusetts: Harvard University Press; 2014.

23. Reeves RV, Howard K. The Parenting Gap. Washington, DC: Center on Children & Families, Brookings Institution; 2013.

24. Black RE, Victora CG, Walker SP, Bhutta ZA, Christian P, de Onis M, et al. Maternal and Child Undernutrition and Overweight in Low-Income and Middle-Income Countries. The Lancet. 2013;382(9890):427–51.

25. Popkin BM, Adair LS, Ng SW. Global Nutrition Transition and the Pandemic of Obesity in Developing Countries. Nutrition Reviews. 2012;70(1):3–21.

26. Holmes J. John Bowlby and Attachment Theory. London; New York, NY: Routledge; 1993.

27. Burtle A, Bezruchka S. Population Health and Paid Parental Leave: What the United States Can Learn from Two Decades of Research. Healthcare. 2016;4(2), 30; doi:10.3390/healthcare4020030.

28. Collins C. Making Motherhood Work: How Women Manage Careers and Caregiving. Princeton: Princeton University Press; 2019.

29. Hart B, Risley TR. Meaningful Differences in the Everyday Experience of Young American Children. Baltimore: P.H. Brookes; 1995.

30. Barrington DS, Adeyemo AA, Rotimi CN. Childhood Family Living Arrangements and Blood Pressure in Black Men: The Howard University Family Study. Hypertension. 2014;63(1):48–53.

31. DeMause L, editor. The History of Childhood. New York, NY: Harper & Row; 1974.

32. Felitti VJ, Anda RF. The Lifelong Effects of Adverse Childhood Experiences. In: Chadwick DL, Alexander R, Giardino AP, Essemio-Jenssen D, Thackeray JD, editors. Chadwick's Child Maltreatment Sexual Abuse and Psychological Maltreatment. Volume 2. Saint Louis, MO: STM Learning; 2014. pp. 203–15.

33. Burke Harris N. The Deepest Well: Healing the Long-Term Effects of Childhood Adversity. Boston: Houghton Mifflin; 2018.

34. Heckman JJ. Promoting Social Mobility. Boston Review. 2012 September/October.

35. Heckman JJ. The Economics of Inequality: The Value of Early Childhood Education. American Educator. 2011;35(1):31–47.

36. Campbell F, Conti G, Heckman JJ, Moon SH, Pinto R, Pungello E, et al. Early Childhood Investments Substantially Boost Adult Health. Science. 2014;343(6178):1478–85.

37. Eckenrode J, Campa M, Luckey DW, Henderson CR, Cole R, Kitzman H, et al. Long-Term Effects of Prenatal and Infancy Nurse Home Visitation on the Life Course of Youths 19-Year Follow-up of a Randomized Trial. Archives of Pediatrics & Adolescent Medicine. 2010;164(1):9–15.

38. Sonchak L. The Impact of WIC on Birth Outcomes: New Evidence from South Carolina. Maternal and Child Health Journal. 2016;20(7):1518–25.

39. Bradbury B, Corak M, Waldfogel J, Washbrook E. Too Many Children Left Behind: the U.S. Achievement Gap in Comparative Perspective. New York, NY: Russell Sage Foundation; 2015.

40. Warren E, Tyagi AW. The Two-Income Trap: Why Middle-Class Mothers and Fathers Are Going Broke. New York, NY: Basic Books; 2003.

41. Public Health Agency of Canada. What Makes Canadians Healthy or Unhealthy?: Government of Canada; 2013 [cited 2013 January 15]. Available from: https://www.canada.ca/en/public-health/services/health-promotion/population-health/what-determines-health/what-makes-canadians-healthy-unhealthy.html.

Chapter 6

Health Inequities

> Equality is getting shoes, equity is getting shoes that fit.
>
> *Naheed Dosani*

It is decidedly unfair and unjust that we Americans don't have the best health when we think we have the best of almost everything in the world. Besides the unfairness of living in a country with so many health issues, there is also the inequity of health outcomes for people within the United States. Consider the unequal health outcomes of groups within the United States that are unfair. Some of us are doing better than others. How do we know that?

When I went to public health school, test scores were posted on a bulletin board identified by student numbers so we could see where we stood in relation to our classmates. At the end of my first year of college in Toronto, one's name and rank in class was published in Canada's largest circulation newspaper. Anyone could see where they stood—a practice which inspired all of us to do our best. While not everyone will face such public display of their rankings, today we are exposed to a dynamic sorting system which illuminates how well we are doing nationally and globally. Income or wealth represents one such ranking. Power represents another ordering. Richer people have more power than poorer ones, despite the poor far outnumbering the rich, and COVID has vastly expanded the gulf between the rich and the poor as the wealth of our nation's richest billionaires increased by $1.2 trillion during the pandemic's first year, while 20,000,000 Americans lost their jobs, and countless others lost their homes, incomes, even their lives.

The higher the income inequality in a society, the bigger the gap between richer and poorer and the steeper the slope of the income health graph. The pitch of that incline is determined by power relationships in a society thus making health a political construct. Here, we take a closer look at the social factors, the gradient, that shape the health we have today.

DOI: 10.4324/9781003315889-7

Social Determinants of Health

Modern-day understandings of the social origins of health began in the 1600s in England where county parish death rates were discovered to be strongly impacted by poverty, poor housing, working conditions, and insecure diets, among others. The industrial revolution during the 19th century in Europe compounded the carnage. Charles Dickens's novels graphically depicted this era's poverty and social stratification. Consider his observation, voiced by Ebenezer Scrooge, in *A Christmas Carol*. "There is nothing on which it is so hard as poverty; and there is nothing it professes to condemn with such severity as the pursuit of wealth!"

By the mid to late nineteenth century, when Dickens was writing, poverty was extreme, but something changed to mitigate the health impacts on the poor. Country mortality rates began falling with public health improvements first in Scandinavia, then England and France. Those health gains were linked to better standards of living and hygiene. Keeping fecal waste separated from food and water produced a critical advance in the quality of life. Less crowding and better ventilation in homes, as well as improved nutrition, benefitted health phenomenally.

Despite these improvements in hygiene, when it comes to medical care the health gradient (poorer people having poorer health) hasn't improved much. Take deaths from measles mentioned in the previous chapter. The big decline occurred before there was an immunization and was due to improved living conditions. Today, where there is universal access to healthcare, poorer people use it more, yet they still have worse health. A good example is in England with its National Health System which provides free medical care to all. Studies of national civil servants doing office work in the Whitehall complex of government buildings in central London found mortality from heart disease varied fourfold among occupational classes, even though they all sat at desks and did not engage in hazardous work. Lower-ranking civil servants smoked more and had higher cholesterol among other risk factors. However, such reasons for having higher death rates explained only a small fraction of the difference. What mattered most was their employment rank, which also reflected their social class in England(1). Another example, in Winnipeg, Canada, was discussed in Chapter 2 where those with less education or lower incomes used more medical care and died younger. Medical care doesn't erase class differences in health outcomes.

Socioeconomic status (SES), where you stand on the ladder that ranks people economically and socially in a society, is the key concept impacting so many health outcomes. SES can be measured in many ways including by how much income you make. Or how much wealth you have. Or your highest educational attainment as in Chapter 5. Or your occupational status. SES measures allow comparisons to others. On the many forms you typically fill out, only a few ask for your income. They may ask you to choose a race, and very likely will ask whether you graduated from high school, or from college or beyond. All these responses are markers of your SES, even if income is not explicitly requested.

In any standard study of a behavior, drug or substance affecting our health scientists must first control for SES. In many studies, the groups we compare are unlikely to all be college graduates or make the same income. So in the analysis we measure a marker for SES and then remove its effect in the study so it has no bearing on the results. If you ask the researchers why they do that, the typical reply is, "without doing that we don't find the effect we are looking for." In other words, researchers have to negate the impact of the hierarchy represented by SES to see if something else has an impact. Logically, the most important component in a health study is SES. This knee-jerk practice is almost never questioned. Yet can we entirely negate the effect of SES? Likely not since so many variables are impacted by SES, but we can at least attenuate its impact.

Over 25 years ago, however, epidemiologists began to not always routinely control their studies for SES. They wanted to see just how important SES really was as a variable. They wanted to see how the distribution of advantages and disadvantages in society reflected its health. Not controlling for SES birthed social epidemiology. Consider social epidemiology as that branch of epidemiology looking at how social structures, institutions and relationships influence health. Therein, you'll discover what needs to be done to improve health.

The phrase "social determinants of health" became more commonly used in 1998 after the publication of *Social Determinants of Health: The Solid Facts*, authored by two visionaries, Richard Wilkinson and Michael Marmot(2). The first textbook in the field, *Social Epidemiology,* appeared in 2000, while a commission of The World Health Organization (WHO) produced a major report on *Social Determinants of Health* (SDOH) in 2008(3, 4). Since then, the phrase has been increasingly used in public health departments around the globe. Yet the term remains mostly unknown to people in the United States.

What are the SDOH? Consider them the non-medical determinants of health, namely, everything besides biomedical care that produces health in a population—"the conditions in which we are born, live, work, and play." Recognizing SDOH represents a scientific revolution in thinking about health.

Americans have been slow to recognize the importance of social determinants. Our leading federal health agency, the Center for Disease Control and Prevention (CDC) highlighted them first in a technical report published in 2011 where they also pointed out that the United States had the highest income inequality of all rich nations. More recently, state and local public health departments have taken the cue to present this specialized material. Until COVID came along, however, there were no cataclysmic events to launch a new direction like the dropping of two atomic bombs on Japan in World

War II that spawned the awareness of nuclear energy, or the 1957 Russian launch of the satellite Sputnik that began the race to the moon. Then in 2020, COVID burst into lives.

One catastrophic event can give us a window into how social determinants shape our survival. Consider those who survived the sinking of the Titanic(5). Sixty percent of those with a first class ticket lived. Forty percent holding second-class passage survived, while only a quarter of third class or crew made it out alive. This gradient, survival depending on which class of ticket you held on the Titanic, is ubiquitous—those in first class have better results on just about any ship or circumstance.

COVID-19 survival similarly patterns Titanic data. Essential workers (the crew), African Americans, and poorer people (third class) have had higher death rates in the United States than those with first class passage in the United States (the richest 10% say). In New York City, the highest death rates have been among those with the lowest income. As discussed in Chapter 3, income inequality is a major factor related to increased deaths in the pandemic.

During the first COVID wave, an increase in income inequality correlated with an increased number of cases across the globe, as well as the finding that poorer people did poorly. While we have seen inequality soar in the United States, we don't yet have good data for the pandemic's impact on inequality across the globe. We expect that changes in income inequality will produce changes in COVID outcomes as we saw in Chapter 3 with Japan as an example where inequality decreased and health improvements soared, and the Soviet Union where the opposite happened.

Socioeconomic gradients can be compared among countries for various health outcomes. As we saw in Chapter 5, having a low birthweight limits health improvements. Studying four English-speaking countries, Australia, Canada, New Zealand and the United States, researchers divided each country into five equal portions (or quintiles) of income to look at what proportion of babies in each are born with low birthweights(6). People in the poorest fifth within the United States have almost two-and-a-half times the proportion of such births compared to the richest fifth. A third more low birthweight babies are born here than for the poorest fifth in England and the gradient is steeper for Blacks in the United States than in England. Another study looking at the chance immigrants to the United States have of delivering a low birthweight baby found the rate was less than for native-born. But the longer immigrants stay in the United States the less the advantage, suggesting something is toxic about living in America(7).

The major 2008 WHO report on SDOH mentioned above had three critical recommendations: (1) improve daily living conditions; (2) tackle the inequitable distribution of power, money, and resources; and (3) measure and understand the problem and assess the impact of action. So let's start by understanding the problem.

Inequity, Inequality, and Disparity

Health disparity is a common U.S. term to describe a difference in health outcomes. Other countries use health inequality and health inequity, terms less commonly used here. Think of inequality as an unfair difference. For example, consider two people, one who was abandoned in early life and now is homeless, and another who grew up in a secure environment and has a home. An inequity is an inequality that can be fixed or remedied. The severe homeless situation in the United States results from government policies beginning in 1980 that cut funding for low-cost housing. That inequality is not only unfair, but it can be remedied

The CDC describes health equity, the brand and process, as "Health equity is achieved when every person has the opportunity to "attain his or her full health potential" and no one is "disadvantaged from achieving this potential because of social position or other socially determined circumstances." But to reach that state of equity, we must fix the problem, but we can't fix something until we understand why it's broken.

Political Determinants of Health

Hawai'i is the healthiest state in the United States with the longest life expectancy and among the lowest mortality rates of all states. The United Health Foundation's 2020 report ranks it number one in health outcomes(8). Hawai'i's Department of Health produced *Chronic Disease Disparities Report 2011: Social Determinants* which includes a key graphic (reproduced below) summarizing their findings on SDOH (Figure 6.1). They distinguish the Downstream "Effects" or *Makai* producing health from the Upstream "Root Causes" or *Mauka*. They illustrate this metaphor with the image of a mountain from which flows a stream that becomes a raging waterfall that turns into a river which empties into the ocean. In the ocean are the Chronic Disease Burdens such as cancer, heart disease, and diabetes. On opposite shores of the river flowing into the ocean are Risk Factors (smoking, physical inactivity, obesity) on the one side and on the other Access to Healthcare (insurance, costs, medical-home). On opposite sides of the impressive waterfall are two text columns. On the one side are Discrimination/Racism, Community Context (Deprivation, Crime, Safety, Housing), Geography/Place, Environment/Pollution, and Poverty. On the other side, you see Education, Employment/Occupation, Risk Markers (race/ethnicity/age), and Income/Wealth. These waterfall elements represent the social determinants. Above that and just below the saddle on the mountain ridge are two lines of text. Lower down you'll find "Social/Economic Conditions" and above that, just below the ridge, are "Political Context and Governance."

This artwork symbolizes almost all you need to know about the priorities of health production. If we want to minimize the chronic disease

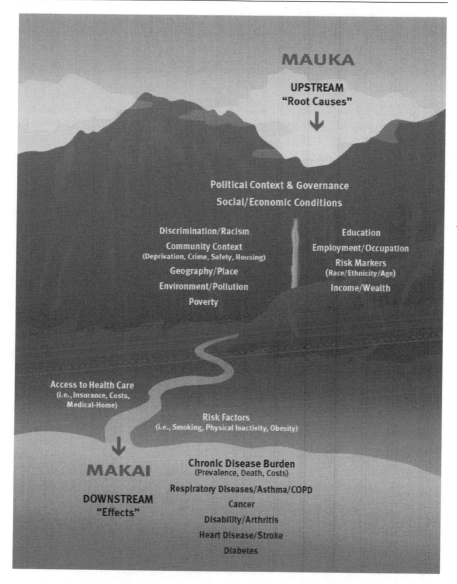

Figure 6.1 Department of Health, Hawai'i's determinants of health graphic(9).

burden, we must look to socioeconomic conditions, and most importantly political contexts and governance. Health results from collective decisions made through the political process. Yet the importance of politics in producing health is rarely mentioned in most discussions of factors that make societies healthier.

Public health's biggest idea was stated by Rudolf Virchow, the father of modern cellular pathology, in 1848(10):

> Medicine is a social science, and politics nothing but medicine at a larger scale.

The federal report, *Healthy People 2030,* does not mention the impact of politics except for suggesting political participation through voting(11). The question is whether the political factors shaping our health are concealed more through incredulity (people don't believe politics matters most for health) than by not telling the truth.

Health Inequities in the United States

Health inequities have a long history in our country, predating even the nation itself. After European contact with North America in 1492 a systematic destruction of the indigenous peoples began through direct violence and intentionally distributing disease vectors to them by giving them blankets from smallpox victims. These blankets sickened and killed large numbers of indigenous people. In Massachusetts during the mid-eighteenth century, Whites were paid a bounty of over 300 pounds for killing and scalping an Indian. Numbers were decimated from more than one hundred million Native Americans (more people than in Europe at that time) to perhaps ten million a hundred years later. Given that health is transmitted inter-generationally, that is from one generation to the next, and recognizing the historical trauma American indigenous have suffered, they have the worst health outcomes in the United States today.

To observe this striking carnage, look at maps of life expectancy in the United States by counties. Figure 6.2 is a map of the United States life expectancy by county for 2019 in greyscale with dark grey being 64.5 years and lightest grey being 91.7 depicting huge geographical health inequalities(12). Striking dark grey patterns stand out for upper Midwest counties housing Indian reservations. We see the coloniality of public health—what happened to indigenous people with colonization. Pine Ridge Indian Reservation in South Dakota has the worst health outcomes in the country, even lower than the Oglala Lakota county where it sits. If that county were a nation, it would rank its health around 140th globally—a massive health inequity. Given this legacy, it is no surprise that American natives have done very poorly in the pandemic.

The other striking pattern of worse health (darker grey) is found in the Mississippi Valley and parts of the southeast and into Appalachia especially West Virginia and neighboring Kentucky where poverty is so prevalent. One can map many other health indicators that show similar patterns. These include common cancers, strokes, heart disease, obesity, diabetes, teen births, infant mortality, low birthweight, pre-term births, smoking, stress, homicides, and mass shootings. Declines in life expectancy show similar distributions with Appalachia and the southeast demonstrating absolute drops in the

US County Life Expectancy 2019

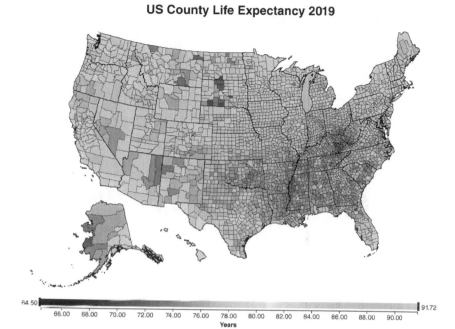

Figure 6.2 Life expectancy, U.S. counties 2019(12).[1]

20 years after 1987. There have been substantial declines in life expectancy for most counties from 2014 to 2019. To observe specific trends go to the IHME website(12) and look at years from 2000 on and for different racial and ethnic groups. One can also look at many other indicators to gauge health inequities.

The next health inequity applies to those of African American descent. Slavery and the impact of racism continue to impact the health of all Americans today, and not only the descendants of slaves. The worst regional health (including Whites) in the United States is in the southeast where slavery predominated. Recall the importance of birth weight as an indicator of adult health. African Americans have the highest rates of low birthweight babies in this country, almost twice as high as Whites, and those rates are increasing. We tend to believe that achieving higher educational status will ameliorate such problems. In 1996, college-educated Black women had a higher proportion of babies born of low birthweight than any other racialized group of any educational status in the United States, higher than Whites not graduating from high school, or Latinx or American Indians(13). An African American woman cannot erase the color of her skin even by attaining the highest level of schooling. Her baby will still have compromised health.

Consider women immigrating to the United States from Africa. Their babies have birthweights comparable to White women and considerably higher than American-born Blacks(14). Why? The socially mediated stress of racism has a profound effect on health outcomes. African women living in the United States have not experienced racism to the degree of American-born Blacks. This advantage deteriorates for subsequent generations that are descendants of African-born Blacks.

The effects of stress are transmitted from one generation to the next through epigenetic means that we will consider in the next chapter. Though we do not have birthweight outcomes for American slaves, we know that one-year-old babies born of slave mothers were very small. Birthweights are transmitted from one generation to the next. If you are a woman born of low birthweight, you are more likely to have a baby of low birthweight. The low birthweights of African Americans today result from the intergenerational transmission since slavery(15). The rates are highest for Blacks in the southeast of the United States, which is an inequality and remediable, thus making it an inequity.

We saw in Chapter 5 that being born with a low birth weight results in lower school test scores suggesting brain development compromise. One reason for Blacks not doing so well in school can be attributed to their high rates of being born with low birth weight. More or better schooling is a good idea but that is a more downstream intervention. Also presented there were impacts of various traumatic events on birth weight.

Recall ACEs or adverse childhood experiences. They are more common among U.S. Blacks, families with low incomes and in regions of higher income inequality. The pandemic has also exacerbated occurrences of ACEs. All these factors limit health gains.

Another large, racialized health outcome are deaths of women from childbirth-related causes, otherwise known as maternal mortality. The United States is one of only a handful of countries that have seen increases in maternal mortality over the last few years(16). African American mothers suffer about three times the chance of dying from childbirth-related causes than other racialized group(17). Maternal mortality has increased with COVID-19. Racism explains part of this tragedy. Another is the substandard medical care that Blacks tend to receive here. These disproportionate rates of maternal mortality among Black women are an inequity. Racism is inextricably linked to poverty and poor health.

Racism

Racism reflects difference plus power. We perceive differences and use power to subjugate. But there are no biological differences underlying race. As significant as race may seem, race is a social construct. There is no way to identify race through genetic differences. From prehistory to the present people migrated and mated producing offspring that do not conform to any racialized category. As a result, there is more genetic difference within races than between them. However, many White Americans believe that African Americans represent a lower class of human flesh. Denying voting rights to U.S. Blacks today reflects one response to their presumed inferiority. Another reason is constraining Black power especially after centuries of discrimination in the United States. The ability to limit the power that Blacks might have through exercising their constitutional rights as voting citizens typifies White privilege, as White communities do not face the same challenges to access polls. Differential sentencing guidelines for cocaine (predominantly used by Whites) and crack cocaine (more common among Blacks) is another example. The ubiquitous surveillance of Blacks in department stores, the heightened abuse of Blacks by police officers, or the constant fears many Whites have when Blacks are living their lives in public spaces, is yet another example.

Racism's forms include personally mediated racism, internalized racism and institutional racism. I depict the internalized version in my teaching by showing a one minute video titled, "Black Doll White Doll." Young African American children are presented with dolls representing the two skin colors. They choose the White doll as better, having internalized the belief that White is better than Black. Such studies began here in the 1930s and have shown consistently similar results(18). The question is how does someone come to internalize one as superior, and the other as inferior?

Consider this gardener's tale(19). The gardener plants flower seeds from two different packages, one for red flowers and the other for pink, in two different soils. One, the red, went into new potting soil and the other into what was used the previous year. The red grows brilliantly. The gardener is impressed by the red flowers and doesn't recognize the soil differences. If a seed from a pink flower is blown into the rich soil, she plucks it out before it can establish itself. Unconscious of how she has differently planted and tended the flowers, she concludes the red are inherently better.

When we talk about racism, what many people think of is personally mediated racism—the blatant discrimination against people of color. Examples include a White crossing the street to avoid a face-to-face encounter with a Black person, store detectives following Blacks in department stores, and police killings of unarmed Blacks.

Institutional or structural racism is more like the gardener not recognizing the soil differences that result in the preferred red flowers. It reflects how society is set up to limit what racialized underdogs can achieve. Let's probe its structural form.

Consider income and wealth inequality in the United States. Historically redlining cordoned off Black communities to limit eligibility for mortgage loans. The home appraisals of Black families are measurably less than those of Whites. Environmental waste and toxins are much more likely to be located in communities of color than in White neighborhoods. And I've already mentioned how financing our schools by property taxes leads to unequal educations. In addition, median (middle) incomes are much lower for Blacks than for Whites. Since 1967 Black incomes as a percentage of Whites are unchanged or have worsened from the bottom fifth to the top brackets. Net worth or wealth differences are much starker. Net Black family worth is around $20,000, meaning they have close to equal amounts of debt to assets with hardly any progress made since the 1980s, while White Americans have seen their net worth double to over $150,000 before COVID(20). This century's median White wealth has increased but Black has not. Consider the gardener in our allegory as the U.S. government who has created these soils.

The pandemic has further widened the gap. Racism's effects on health are additive to those of inequality and historical trauma. Besides the intergenerational transmission of slavery trauma to explain why American Blacks having worse health today, Arline Geronimus' coined "weathering" as the cumulative stresses as people age(21). Blacks experience more weathering so as we will see in the next chapter they have more wear and tear on their bodies.

Fortunately, there had been some progress in reducing Black–White health differences. The Black-White life expectancy gap had been decreasing since the 1950s although improvements stagnated in the last decade. In 1990, the gap was 7 years dropping to 3.4 years in 2014(22). Recall the Black White adult mortality trends in Chapter 4. COVID-19 has produced striking declines in Black life expectancy from almost 75 years in 2019 to 71.8 in 2020(23). During that same year White life expectancy decreased a little over a year to 77.6 thereby widening the Black–White gap and eradicating decades of progress. Reasons include the inability to work from home, lack of access to COVID testing and vaccines and vaccine hesitancy resulting from centuries of medical and public health biases perpetrated onto Black bodies—a form of social murder.

More Health Inequities

Racism against Blacks is not the only inequity that impacts health. The Latinx (also called Hispanic and Latino) present a special case. Before COVID came along, Latinx had better health than non-Latinx Whites, as measured by life expectancy, infant mortality and other benchmarks(24). But Latinx, in general, are poorer than Whites. Their better outcomes have been known for over thirty years and labeled as the epidemiological or Hispanic or Latino paradox(25). Reasons considered include the healthy migrant effect (only those with good health come to the United States), the salmon hypothesis (the sick go home to die), and cultural or social factors. Studies of the first two do not show a big effect(26, 27). My personal experience in the emergency department was that I never saw a lone Latinx patient. I saw a large group of people crowded around a stretcher, and in the middle was the patient while the rest were family members and friends who came to support that person. Meanwhile in the next bed was a White man moaning alone. The strong social support that is inherent in their culture produces a profound health benefit.

The health benefits of friends and social support have been studied for over 40 years and found to greatly impact mortality. Lack of such social solidarity increases death rates far more than personal behaviors such as smoking, over-eating, not exercising, not seeing your doctor and many others(28).

The socioeconomic and health gradient is less steep for Latinx, compared to Whites. The longer Latinx live here, or the further they live from their point of entry to the United States, the closer their health outcomes converge to those of non-Latinx Whites. At least part of that relative decline in health advantage comes from loss of their traditional supportive culture.

Along with Blacks, Latinx have suffered disproportionate COVID deaths. The largest drop in life expectancy from 2019 to 2020 was for Latinx males, followed by Black males, then Black women, then Latinx females(23). The smallest drop was for non-Latinx male and female Whites. The drop in years for Latinx men was almost three times that for White males. The strong Latinx social support system did not protect them from the essential work they had to do to support their families. They were exposed more to SARS-CoV-2 in proportion to their numbers. The most vulnerable were poorer people. Even so, Latinx Americans still had higher life expectancies than Whites (1.2 more years over Whites in 2020), maintaining the health benefits they enjoy.

Sexual orientation differences, LGBTQIA+ (Lesbian, Gay, Bisexual, Transgender, Queer, Indeterminant (or Intersex), Asexual, and others), also demonstrate health inequities that are similar to racism's prejudice and dis-crimination. Gender identity reflects how you perceive your own gender, while sexual identity is who you have sex with (i.e., are attracted to). In the last decade national surveys estimate close to 4% of people in the United States identify as LGB with half of those as Bisexual—likely underestimates.

Homosexuality is still greatly stigmatized in the United States even though a 2015 Supreme Court decision allows same-sex marriages, and despite the fact that homosexuality is universal among primates—who we are. Transgender acceptance is low but increasing slowly in rich nations. LGBT people suffer discrimination at school and in employment status, earnings, and job advance-ment. Acceptability of homosexuality is greater among women, younger people, those more educated (reflecting the socioeconomic gradient) and people living in urban areas.

LGBTQ have worse health outcomes(29). These likely include higher mor-tality rates, more ACEs, worse mental health, lower life satisfaction, higher substance use, and problematic access to medical care(30). They also suffer intense discrimination. Gays can still be executed in some countries. Health inequities abound for LGBTQ. Yet what about male–female health differences?

In vertebrates, males die before females. The human female advantage begins at birth with fewer babies dying in the first year of life(31, 32). This most pre-dictable pattern of mortality has been observed at all ages in rich countries during the last century, and it has been reported as far back as 1750. The gender gap in survival is largest in Russia. A host of reasons have been offered including biological advantages, gene differences, social benefits, among oth-ers. Warfare also plays a role. Sri Lankan adult women have lower mortality than American women but the civil war there has produced the opposite for men. Male competition for mates plays a role at least in wild animals.

Genetic differences matter. Men have an X chromosome deficiency disorder. Y chromosomes (present in men) have about 100 genes while the X chromosome has ten-plus times more. Women have two X chromosomes so if a mutation occurs in one that may not benefit health, the other chromosome might be expressed to avoid deterioration, giving women an advantage over men. There are also hormonal advantages. Testosterone may limit health in men, while estrogen and oxytocin secretion may benefit women's health. Pregnancy and delivery are more hazardous at older ages, but menopause may limit these perils.

The female life expectancy advantage in the United States has varied from 6 to 7 years until the late 1990s when it decreased to about 5 years. There was a correlation with state income inequality where more unequal states had higher sex differences in life expectancy, namely, women lived longer in these unequal states. Reasons include greater female resilience under economic adversity than males (they can handle inequality better) and men being traditionally the income earners (having more stress in higher gap states).

Life expectancy variations with income follow a predictable pattern. When we divide the United States into fifths of incomes and look at life expectancy trends, we find that between 1980 and 2010 life expectancy for men stagnated for the poorest fifth. The richest fifth saw striking gains, and correspondingly less for the other three fifths by income with hardly any for the second lowest fifth(33). The richest 1% of American men now live 15 years longer than the poorest 1%. As the map above illustrates, where you live matters too, for example, you're likely to live longer in New York City compared to Detroit. For women the trends were even starker. Only the richest fifth saw gains in life expectancy while the bottom four-fifths saw declines over that 30-year period.

These many inequities suggest that something is happening during our lives that lead us to live shorter or longer lives, depending on our social status. But recall my point that our health is largely determined at birth. Is our poor health in the United States something that results from conditions earlier in life or later?

In the early 1950s, both American men and women had the best chances of surviving to age 50 compared to other rich nations. Consistent with gender differences, men had higher mortality to age 50 than women but American men did better than those in other nations. This health advantage among countries deteriorated so that by 1990 for women and by 2004 for men, those in all the other rich nations had lower mortality than Americans. The chances of dying early in life declined in America but like so many other health indicators, it declined faster in other countries. Something significant was affecting mortality in the first half of life for Americans more than for those in other rich countries. That something included rising income inequality and the lack of support for early life. But what about after age 50?

Life expectancy can be calculated at any age. If we take how many years of life are left when someone reaches age 50, we can look at trends from 1955 to the present to illustrate patterns(34). For Australia, France, Japan, Spain and the United States, we find that in 1955 fifty-year-old American women had the most years of life to look forward to while Japanese women had the least(35). Yet Japanese women raced ahead of us and by 1980 were ahead of all other countries. In contrast, the United States saw solid improvements in life expectancy at age 50 until 1980 after which our improvements began falling behind the others, whereas men did not see their years left at age 50 worsening until more recently. The relative decline in health for American women, in contrast to other nations, can be attributed to the increasing expectations placed on them. As women entered the job market in other rich nations, they received more support from their governments, including paid maternal leave, smaller gender pay gaps, and government support including free education at all levels from preschool on. In the United States, however, that support has not been forthcoming, so that by age 50, women in the United States are expected to not only have a valued career, but also be loving wives, attentive mothers, excellent homemakers, have the physique of an athlete, and the looks of a supermodel. Expectations for men, however, have remained unchanged over this time period. It's no wonder women who reach the age of 50 in the United States no longer fare as well as their counterparts in other rich nations (Figure 6.3). These mortality differences represent health inequities for those of us living in the United States. They can be fixed, however.

Consider the boundary between older and younger ages. Recent analysis of mortality data among rich nations has demonstrated what are called deaths of despair in the United States. Mortality from 1990 to 2015 among Americans aged 45 to 54, was compared with the same age range of those in Australia,

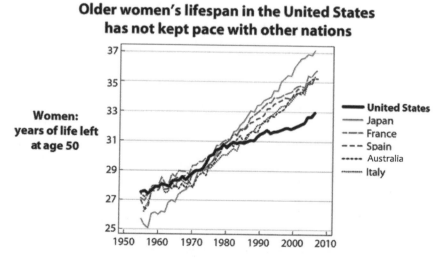

Figure 6.3 Female life expectancy at age 50 trends (1955–2007), six rich nations(35).

Canada, France, Germany, Sweden, and the United Kingdom. They show dramatic differences. Mortality declined over that period for those in the other nations but not for U.S. Whites.

Deaths from drugs, alcohol issues and suicides increased markedly over the same time period for U.S. Whites compared to the other countries. This rise was not seen with African Americans, Latinx or Asian-Pacific Islanders in the United States. American Whites reaching the prime of their lives had expected to achieve the American Dream, namely, to become rich. Consistent with rising income and wealth inequality this group has not seen the betterment of their lives, and many succumb through drugs and suicide(36).

There are more firearms than people in the United States. States with higher rates of gun ownership appear to have higher suicide rates. Research had been hampered by the National Rifle Association (NRA) which lobbies Congress to not fund such studies. The pattern may be strongest for those born in 1970 and aged 45 to 54 with lower incomes or lower education levels. There was no suicide difference for those born in 1945. Suicide rates in other countries with credible data have been falling since 2000. Consistent with our falling health status and high stress levels, however, suicide is rising in America.

We have also seen a drug-induced overdose epidemic over the last few decades here. People in this country now consume around three-quarters of the world's opioids. Opioids have been used for 5000 years, but they are now synthesized and routinely prescribed for pain relief, often for disorders easily treated with over-the-counter analgesics. The result has been a surge in opioid addiction.

Our opioid mortality epidemic stems from the painful state of living in America—we suffer great social pain. People seek relief from this pain in various ways including prescription opioids and those available elsewhere. Many opioids we consume illicitly have considerable amounts of very potent fentanyl. Too much of an opioid stops breathing, causing death. I saw many patients whose respiratory function had failed as a result of such drugs. I had a Rule of Fours in the emergency department: you can survive 4 minutes without air, 4 days without water and 4 weeks without food. If you were not breathing, that means you had only four minutes to live, so I had to act quickly.

Deaths from such drug overdoses are estimated to be more than half a million since their use increased over the last half century. They rose to over 93,000 in 2020(37). The overdose deaths in 2020 are over four times the gun deaths that year.

Opioids were heavily marketed by Big Pharma over the last 30 years, contributing to this rise in drug addiction and deaths—and a rise in lawsuits against Big Pharma. Those drug companies are now settling to avoid more lawsuits. The heyday of opioid over-prescribing by doctors has thankfully passed.

Those with social pain often self-medicate with alcohol and marijuana. Marijuana has been used as a recreational drug and to treat health issues for millennia. It has a better safety profile than opioids and alcohol. No matter how much is consumed, it will not stop the heart or respiratory system. Nonetheless, despite being prohibited at the federal level since 1937, and classed with heroin, legal use among United States has risen. But the prohibition of cannabis has branded it with a social stigma among many, while alcohol remains socially acceptable. As a result, alcohol use remains rampant, and alcohol abuse and addiction remain especially high among those living with social pain.

COVID has produced more of this social pain so people medicate themselves. Social media have been flooded with jokes, memes and confessions of people drinking more during the pandemic. We do not yet have statistics on the rise in drug-related injuries and deaths to assess the impact of COVID on alcohol use, but we can expect to find disturbing data.

These political foundations of our health inequities are treated as if they are the hysteria of liberals seeking to deprive conservatives of their "rights," whether that be the right not to wear a mask, the right not to get a vaccine, the right to buy as many guns as possible, and the like. Yet liberal policies are more likely to extend our lives.

An important study looked at state life expectancy from 1958 to 2017 stratified by how liberal the state policies were(38). Liberal policies include those regarding abortion, civil rights, criminal justice, education, gun control, health and welfare, housing, labor, LGBTQ rights, progressive tax rates and voting among others. The more liberal the state policies the higher the life expectancy gain over that almost 60 year period. Consider Oklahoma and Connecticut, two states that had the same life expectancy in 1958. By 2017, Connecticut had an almost seven year greater lifespan related to its more liberal governmental policies. This finding supports the political context and governance voiced by the health department in Hawai'i as the most upstream factor affecting health.

How a county voted for U.S. president in elections from 2001 to 2019 was associated with mortality. Republican voting counties had higher mortality rates than counties voting Democratic, and the death gap from 2001 to 2019 increased markedly. Over that time period for Blacks the mortality gap didn't change much by voting status, while for Whites it increased. For Latinx there was almost no difference in mortality by voting status. Consistent with what we have already said, Latinx had the lowest mortality rates.

The political affiliation of U.S. state governors impacts COVID-19 parameters. Initially, Republican-led states had better outcomes. For the first part of 2020 the initial port of entry for the SARS-CoV-2 virus was mostly in Democrat-led states—the coastal states, where international travel was most common. Since June 2020, however, Democrat-led states have decreased cases, with more testing and fewer deaths than Republican-led states. As the pandemic became widespread, Republican-led states were less likely to adopt protective measures, such as physical distancing, masking and stay at home orders, to contain the virus(39). There are similar findings at the county level. Immunization policies follow these patterns. More liberal policies benefit health outcomes.

Geographers speak of the sense of place. Consider criminal justice policies. Living in a county with high incarceration rates is associated with lower birthweight. According to a 2021 study, if you live in a New York state census tract (much smaller than a county) where many have been imprisoned, that tract will have lower life expectancy(40). Even after adjusting for poverty and racial makeup, there remains a two-year gap. Recall from Chapter 4 that we house a quarter of the world's prisoners. Almost one of every hundred Americans is behind bars. Decarceration or reducing our prison population would improve our health.

Conclusion

As this discussion of health inequities shows, to fix the problem, we must first understand that there is a problem. We are then tasked with addressing the root cause of the problem, not hammering away at something else just because the cause of the problem is complex. Just pushing the remote control when it is broken will not fix the TV, anymore than declaring our healthcare system is fine—or saying our unequal society is equal—will repair the health production machine.

But inequity alone is not the only factor to be addressed. In Chapter 3, we discussed criteria for saying something causes something else based on the 1964 Surgeon General's report on smoking and health. We inferred that causality would be established. The missing link requires a discussion of biology. Our biology is associated with inequality and poverty because that combination produces much stress. In the next chapter, we explore the biology of stress to show how societal inequality can and does permeate and damage our bodies, lingering as a silent and invisible killer we come to normalize as the human condition.

Questions to Consider and Discuss

1. How can we gain traction for the importance of politics in health production?
2. Why is so little attention paid to the strong influence of social factors, friendships and networks, on health?

Note

1. Figure 6.2 life expectancies in a few areas of the United States can be misinterpreted because of a number of islands being close together that appear dark in the map. Reference 12 below has the map in color that can be enlarged to show accurate life expectancies for areas in the Pacific Northwest inside Puget Sound, regions of the Chesapeake near Washington D.C. and further north up the Atlantic coast.

References

1. Rose G, Marmot MG. Social Class and Coronary Heart Disease. British Heart Journal. 1981;45:13–9.
2. Wilkinson R, Marmot M, editors. Social Determinants of Health: The Solid Facts. 2nd edition. Copenhagen: World Health Organization Regional Office for Europe; 2003.
3. Berkman LF, Kawachi I, Glymour MM, editors. Social Epidemiology. New York, NY: Oxford University Press; 2014.
4. WHO. Closing the Gap in a Generation: Health Equity Through Action on the Social Determinants of Health. Final Report of the Commission on the Social Determinants of Health. Geneva: World Health Organization; 2008.

5. Hall W. Social Class and Survival on the S.S. Titanic. Social Science & Medicine 1986; 22(6):687–90.

6. Martinson ML, Reichman NE. Socioeconomic Inequalities in Low Birth Weight in the United States, the United Kingdom, Canada, and Australia. American Journal of Public Health. 2016;106(4):748–54.

7. Martinson ML, Tienda M, Teitler JO. Low Birthweight Among Immigrants in Australia, the United Kingdom, and the United States. Social Science & Medicine. 2017;194:168–76.

8. United Health Foundation. America's Health Rankings. Minnetonka, MN: United Health Foundation; 2020.

9. Pobutsky A, Bradbury EW, Tomiyasu D. Chronic Disease Disparities Report 2011: Social Determinants. Honolulu: Hawai'i State Department of Health: Chronic Disease Management and Control Branch; 2011.

10. Mackenbach JP. Politics Is Nothing but Medicine at a Larger Scale: Reflections on Public Health's Biggest Idea. Journal of Epidemiology and Community Health. 2009;63(3):181–4.

11. Office of Disease Prevention and Health Promotion. Healthy People 2030: Building a Healthier Future for All: UI.S. Department of Health and Human Services; 2020 [August 25, 2022] Available from: https://health.gov/healthypeople.

12. Institute for Health Metrics and Evaluation. US Health Map | Viz Hub Seattle University of Washington; 2021 [August 25, 2022] Available from: https://vizhub.healthdata.org/subnational/usa.

13. National Center for Health Statistics. Health, United States, 1998 With Socioeconoic Status and Health Chartbook. Hyattsville: Maryland: National Center for Health Statistics; 1998.

14. David RJ, Collins JW. Differing Birth Weight Among Infants of U.S.-Born Blacks, African-Born Blacks, and U.S.-Born Whites. New England Journal of Medicine. 1997;337(17): 1209–14.

15. Jasienska G. Low Birth Weight of Contemporary African Americans: An Intergenerational Effect of Slavery? American Journal of Human Biology. 2009;21(1):16–24.

16. Kassebaum NJ, Bertozzi-Villa A, Coggeshall MS, Shackelford KA, Steiner C, Heuton KR, et al. Global, Regional, and National Levels and Causes of Maternal Mortality During 1990–2013: A Systematic Analysis for the Global Burden of Disease Study 2013. The Lancet. 2014;384(9947):980–1004.

17. Hoyert DL. Maternal mortality Rates in the United States 2020. NCHS Health E-Stats. 2022.

18. Bergner G. Black Children, White Preference: Brown v. Board, the Doll Tests, and the Politics of Self-Esteem. American Quarterly. 2009;61(2):299–332.

19. Jones CP. Levels of Racism: A Theoretic Framework and a Gardener's Tale. American Journal of Public Health. 2000;90(8):1212–5.

20. Weller C, Roberts L. Eliminating the Black-White Wealth Gap Is a Generational Challenge Washington, D.C.: Center for American Progress; 2021 [cited 2021 March 19]. Available from: https://www.americanprogress.org/article/eliminating-black-white-wealth-gap-generational-challenge/.

21. Geronimus AT, Hicken M, Keene D, Bound J. "Weathering" and Age Patterns of Allostatic Load Scores Among Blacks and Whites in the United States. American Journal of Public Health. 2006;96(5):826–33.

22. National Center for Health Statistics. Health, United States, 2015 With Special Feature on Racial and Ethnic Health Disparities. Hyattsville, MD: US Health and Human Services, Centers for Disease Control; 2016.

23. Arias E, Tejada-Vera B, Ahmad F, Kochanek KD Provisional Life Expectancy Estimates for 2020. National Vital Statistics System: Vital Statistics Rapid Release. 2021.

24. National Center for Health Statistics. Health, United States, 2019. Hyattsville, MD: US Health and Human Services, Centers for Disease Control; 2021.

25. Ruiz JM, Steffen P, Smith TB. Hispanic Mortality Paradox: A Systematic Review and Meta-Analysis of the Longitudinal Literature. American Journal of Public Health. 2013; 103(3):e52–e60.

26. Abraído-Lanza AF, Mendoza-Grey S, Flórez KR. A Commentary on the Latin American Paradox. JAMA Network Open. 2020;3(2):e1921165.

27. Chen Y, Freedman ND, Rodriquez EJ, Shiels MS, Napoles AM, Withrow DR, et al. Trends in Premature Deaths Among Adults in the United States and Latin America. JAMA Network Open. 2020;3(2):e1921085-e.

28. Holt-Lunstad J, Smith TB, Layton JB. Social Relationships and Mortality Risk: A Meta-Analytic Review. PLoS Med. 2010;7(7):e1000316.

29. Graham R, Berkowitz B, Blum R, Bockting W, Bradford J, de Vries B, et al. The Health of Lesbian, Gay, Bisexual, and Transgender People: Building a Foundation for Better Understanding. Washington, DC: Institute of Medicine; 2011. pp. 89–139.

30. Zeeman L, Sherriff N, Browne K, McGlynn N, Mirandola M, Gios L, et al. A Review of Lesbian, Gay, Bisexual, Trans and Intersex (LGBTI) Health and Healthcare Inequalities. Eur J Public Health. 2019;29(5):974–80.

31. Finch CE. The Biology of Human Longevity: Inflammation, Nutrition, and Aging in the Evolution of Life Spans. Burlington, MA: Academic Press; 2007.

32. Oksuzyan A, Gumà J, Doblhammer G. Sex Differences in Health and Survival. In: Doblhammer G, Gumà J, editors. A Demographic Perspective on Gender, Family and Health in Europe: Cham, Switzerland: Springer; 2018. pp. 65–100.

33. National Academies of Sciences Engineering and Medicine. The Growing Gap in Life Expectancy by Income Implications for Federal Programs and Policy Responses. Washington, D.C.: National Academies Press; 2015.

34. Crimmins EM, Preston SH, Cohen B. National Research Council. Panel on Understanding Divergent Trends in Longevity in High-Income C. International Differences in Mortality at Older Ages: Dimensions and Sources. Washington, D.C: National Academies Press; 2010.

35. Glei DA, Meslé F, Vallin J. Diverging Trends in Life Expectancy at Age 50: A Look at Causes of Death. In: Crimmins EM, Preston SH, Cohen B, editors. International Differences in Mortality at Older Ages: Dimensions and Sources. Washington, D.C.: National Academies Press; 2010. p. 17–67.

36. Case A, Deaton A. Deaths of Despair and the Future of Capitalism. Princeton: Princeton University Press; 2020.

37. Ahmad F, Rossen L, Suitton P. Provisional Drug Overdose Death Counts. Washington, D.C.: National Center for Health Statistics; 2021.

38. Montez JK, Beckfield J, Cooney JK, Grumbach JM, Hayward MD, Koytak HZ, et al. US State Policies, Politics, and Life Expectancy. The Milbank Quarterly. 2020;98(3):1–34.

39. Neelon B, Mutiso F, Mueller NT, Pearce JL, Benjamin-Neelon SE. Associations between Governor Political Affiliation and COVID-19 Cases, Deaths, and Testing in the US. American Journal of Preventive Medicine. 2021;61(1):115–9.

40. Holaday LW, Howell B, Thompson K, Cramer L, Wang EA-h. Association of Census Tract-Level Incarceration Rate and Life Expectancy in New York State. Journal of Epidemiology and Community Health. 2021;75(10):1019.

Chapter 7

Stress Is the Killer

If you want to increase your chances of avoiding stress-related diseases, make sure you don't inadvertently allow yourself to be born poor.

Robert Sapolsky, Why Zebras Don't Get Ulcers(1)

We have seen that being poor, especially in early life, results in poor health throughout adult life. If you are born poor, you're not necessarily doomed to be unhealthy; your low socioeconomic status simply decreases the odds that your health will turn out fine. The critical fact to keep in mind is that the poor tend to have worse biological factors affecting their health than the wealthy. The focus on the poor is another way of looking at the steepness of the socioeconomic gradient and health. Having poor people in one's society compromises everyone's health—including their biology. Stress is the mechanism that produces such outcomes.

The Stress Response

Humans have a natural stress response. It's a product of evolution, a mechanism that causes us to deal with deadly situations. I learned this lesson in 1975 when I was hiking behind my remote Nepal home and inadvertently disturbed a Himalayan Brown Bear. One glimpse of the growling creature had me running as fast as I could in the opposite direction. Panting, my lungs rushed the necessary oxygen—already in short supply at the 11,000 foot altitude— to my red blood cells, which were sped up through my circulatory system by my pounding heart which pumped blood furiously to my muscles as I fled, the growling bear close behind. I didn't dare turn around to look until after I could no longer hear the bear's terrifying snarl. Finally, when all was quiet, I sat down, felt my palpitating heart slowing down and my breathing becoming calmer, while my sweat began to chill me in the cold high-altitude air. This instinctive automatic flight reaction may have saved my life. And it all happened without my having to think about what to do.

Having such a rapid response to a serious situation can be lifesaving. We wouldn't be here as a species if, faced with a charging animal, we had to stop

DOI: 10.4324/9781003315889-8

and ponder whether it was a serious threat. Stress, therefore, plays an important role in human survival. But most of the stress we face daily is the sort that does more to threaten our survival than to extend it.

There was no Nepali word for stress in Nepal before the 1970s. Life was hard, but they knew no other way. I didn't see such stress responses then that I saw in the United States. They didn't have problems sleeping (I slept on the floor with many Nepalis in their one-room home), or displays of fidgeting, or signs of muscle tension and almost no high blood pressure. Living in a remote region when there was no mail or electricity available, nor much contact with the outside world, days came and went. The nightly and orderly progression of the constellations and crop cycles marked the yearly passage of seasons. For the agro-pastoralists who lived there, life wasn't stressful, it was just normal hard work. The Nepali word "ee-stress," along with the word tension, only came into use in urban society as it modernized in the 1980s. Prior to that, the concept was unheard of. Now the concept of stress has become ubiquitous in most of the world.

Stress was first described in 1914 by Harvard physiologist Walter Cannon to portray the fight or flight response. In the 1950s, Hans Selye applied the term to the general adaptation syndrome which explained the body's response to demands placed on it.

Curiously, Selye's research was partly funded by the tobacco industry, raising the question whether the concept of stress was, in part, popularized to suggest a problem their product could resolve—namely, you have stress, but our cigarettes can calm you. It is no coincidence that many of the early tobacco advertisements featured medical doctors recommending cigarettes to calm the nerves and alleviate stress. Now, over half a century later, we know that tobacco may alleviate stress, but in so doing there is a high chance it will kill us. What is less known is how deadly stress itself can be in having a similar impact on our health.[1]

When we are exposed to stressors, our bodies produce the stress response. Acute stress results in the fight or flight reaction. This reaction, however, is a short-term phenomenon. It gets us out of trouble and saves lives. The real culprit is chronic stress, the cumulative load of minor or day-to-day stresses that lead to long-term health consequences. Chronic stress can also result from a single focal stress that continues to be experienced long after the situational threat has passed. Psychological stress, a major part of chronic stress today, comes from demands of the environment that exceed one's mental adaptive capacity. Psychosocial stress is imposed on a society by various forces that are common today. Such stress can result in anxiety disorders, panic attacks and other mental illness conditions.

In this chapter, we'll consider what acute stressors do in our bodies, what chronic stress is (in its various forms), and what chronic stress does to our health. We may have some control over these chronic stressors, but this control pales in comparison to what must be achieved in society before we are able to alleviate stressors on a broader level. We will come to see that rather than being life-savers as in the past, the chronic stress that we are exposed to now, especially beginning in early life, produces not only so many of the chronic diseases that will potentially afflict us (if they haven't already), but also many other negative outcomes that we face in today's world. But has it always been like this? Let's think about what stress has been like for humans from prehistory on.

Human Stress from Prehistory to Modern Times

Signs of human stress have been found in bones from unearthed skeletons. These stressors increased with agriculture, as health declined for reasons discussed in Chapter 4.[2] As we've become more sedentary with the transition from gathering and hunting our food, to growing it, we've become less healthy. Few of us produce our food today. Our changing technology has enabled us to shift how we feed ourselves by not having to prepare food. We've created social stratification with unequal access to the food and resources we need to survive. This inequality escalates stress. Over the last couple of centuries, the rising standard of living across the world, together with hygiene improvements and the eventual development of medical care, have improved health. This progress has not been shared equally among both rich and poor, however, partly because forms of stress vary among human classes.

Rising economic inequality leads to more chronic stress. Stress also includes various forms of discrimination, including racism. Ask an African American how often they experience discrimination. Many will say "constantly." Racism has a significant effect on experienced stress, and its reach is not limited to people of color. Racism puts stress on White people, too. In the United States, those states with more overt racism have worse health outcomes for Whites as well as Blacks there. The highest levels of stress in the USA are in the southeastern states where more African Americans live, but the stress of living with racism affects Whites there too. This is consistent with the map of life expectancy in the previous chapter. Both Whites and African Americans, have more obesity there and biomarkers of inflammation, discussed below, are higher there. Adverse health-related behaviors are greater there for both. As we saw in Chapter 6, those states are also the ones with the least socially beneficial expenditure by governments, which is another important reason why health for those living in the southeast states is poor.

Stress also stratifies by class(2). Two forms of class distinctions are by wealth and power. Poorer Americans have considerably more stress than richer Americans who have many ways of buying stress relief: vacation homes, private jets to take them anywhere and staff and advisors to take care of almost any problem. Some have both power and wealth while others, such as the current U.S. president, Joe Biden, have considerable power though not that much wealth. Karl Marx would add a third form of class distinction, employer–employee issues. Employers create a great deal of job stress for their workers.

In our COVIDian era, even doctors in the United States face considerable stress despite having substantial incomes. American women report twice as much stress as men, likely for similar reasons presented in Chapter 6 when looking at years left to live after age 50. Women do much more unpaid work than men also accounting for increased stress.

There are fewer studies focused on discrimination toward LGBTQ individuals, but the results suggest similar effects. Such people tend to be discriminated against and bullied as teens then later develop higher blood pressure and other markers of stress. America has more poverty than other rich nations but even though the reader may not consider herself or himself to be poor, our collective deprivation impacts those reading this book regardless of SES.

In December 2017, the Gallup Poll found eight out of every ten adults in the United States felt stressed every day. In one worldwide report, Americans ranked fifth among 151 countries reporting high stress levels(3). No U.S. city ranks among the ten least stressed cities in the world. Such indicators of stress come from self-reports and are consistent with other markers of stress. Not all stress is negative, however. Some of it is positive.

Some of us actively seek out acute stress that can bring joy or satisfaction, such as rock climbing, skydiving, or white-water rafting. Ultramarathoners stress themselves out for days, as do those engaging in mountain climbing expeditions lasting a month or more. One self-help book titled, *The Joy of Stress,* advises how to make stress work for you(4). Good or positive stress is the type of stress you can variously control and derive personal benefits from. Stress you control can prime your brain and body, allowing you to function at your best. I sought out mountain climbing in my early 20's because I enjoyed that kind of stress which helped me feel competent. I accepted the possibility of dying in major mountains that seemed the most magnificent cathedrals and temples in the world. The positive stress that came of climbing mountains calmed me. There are many types of positive stresses that are good for us. Consider athletic competitions or learning a new skill or steps you take to achieve a worthwhile goal you have set. The stress you feel in striving toward your goals is constructive stress. It propels you to achieve your dreams.

Without positive stress, boredom sets in and we become vegetables. Life is not worth living if we do not experience any stress. Our challenge is to find the right balance. We want just enough positive stress and as little negative stress as possible.

Today's stress is different than the hardships of the past. One would think life should be much easier now than it was a few hundred years ago. Pre-COVID some people could travel to almost anywhere on the planet at a moment's notice. Technological advances enable us to do so much at the push of a button or click of a mouse. Ironically, however, as technology has eased our stress in a multitude of ways, it has at the same time intensified it by other means. Many of us today are mouse workers, typing away on our laptops in unfulfilling work. We expect instantaneous results from our computers and engage in social media that makes us hypervigilant in pursuit of virtual interactions. Yet social media has added to our sense of inequality as we compare our lives to how others present theirs on the internet.

Economic inequality leads to the act of pushing those beneath you further down in the workplace and elsewhere in our lives. Such displaced aggression is a reaction to the increasing economic inequality today(5). In more equal societies, we are more likely to cooperate. There, relationships are those of friendship, support, and solidarity, which are less stressful and more beneficial. In more unequal societies, we reserve our civility for those on a similar level to ours in the socioeconomic hierarchy. We envy the power of those above us, our bosses say, while we suppress any visible or vocal resentment toward them (except, perhaps, anonymously on social media) to avoid angering our superiors. As we do so, we often feel shame.

Shame is the social anxiety that inequality produces and may be our primary social emotion(6). The sense of shame makes us not like ourselves. Feeling shame may imply we are not lovable. Shame and pride emerge from how we are seen in each other's eyes and are key to understanding the experience of poverty. Recall Adam Smith's 1759 concept of not being poor, namely, not wanting to feel ashamed in public. Having pride in public is the fundamental aspect of not being poor. As also noted in Chapter 3, George Bernard Shaw suggested we respond to inequality by putting down those below us. Such dominance and submission behaviors drive much of our lives.

Self-esteem and self-respect are valued concepts in individualistic positivist modern psychology. When we feel we are being evaluated by others, we pretend we are better. This evaluative stress, how others see us, leads to self-enhancement or feeling better than others.

Greater gestures and symbols of self-enhancement are seen in countries with more economic inequality. If we believe we are special, we reason, then perhaps we will be special. We now spend more money on clothes, cars, recreational equipment, than ever (even adjusted for inflation). We live in much larger houses than we did fifty years ago despite families being much smaller now. We buy the newest phones when the phones we bought a year ago have more computer power than took us to the moon. We enculturate our children, marking their superiority to their peers, by way of how we dress them (and how much money we spend dressing them), the toys we buy for them, the pursuit of the best preschools, giving our children an edge to get into the best Ivy League schools, and other status magnifiers.

Then there is social media, a technological enhancement, which is supposedly there to help us do just that—boost our status—but it may work to counter our efforts, as we ultimately can never look or feel quite good enough there. Another "friend" will always have more signs of status in social media forums: more "friends" or followers, more "likes" on their photos, and so on.

Stress is a primary feature of this culture of inequality as we react with submission to some and dominance toward others. Today, despite all our modern "conveniences," we find people constantly talking about stress and how it affects their lives.

Stress Is the 21st-Century Tobacco

"Stress is the 21st century tobacco," was a comment a Seattle cardiologist once made that captures the direction our nation is heading. Smoking, which we know to be bad for us, has declined considerably in the United States, while stress has replaced this hazard. Yet the healthcare professions have mostly not considered human stress as a major cause of poor health. The stress that pervades our lives is like the invisible gas of economic inequality that we live with; it's something that causes much illness and suffering, but many of us are oblivious to this scourge. We see that those lower down the economic ladder face much more stress and will suffer its dire consequences more than those who have more economic security.

COVID-19 has further increased our stress(7). Much media attention during the pandemic has focused on the anxiety we suffer from the pandemic with lockdowns, social isolation, economic crises, parenting while schools are virtual, and fear of falling ill. Many can't cope with this stress. Self-medication such as increasing drinking and opioid use, as well as other drugs, have resulted in record drug overdose deaths. Such stress is additive to what has become normal stress in our societies and together they produce an astonishing amount of poor health outcomes in the United States and other nations. Yet during the pandemic, the United States has not supported its workers to the extent of other rich countries. What happens in our body when we are so chronically stressed?

How Stress Affects the Body

Recall my encounter with a Himalayan Brown Bear. When the brain detects a threat—typically through the sound, touch and sight senses—the brain's amygdala sends a signal to the nearby command center, the hypothalamus, which orchestrates a cascade of responses. One mechanism is carried out through the autonomic nervous system. A part of the autonomic nervous system, the sympathetic nervous system, triggers the response by priming the cardiovascular system to increase heart, lung, and vascular activity to get oxygen and nutrients to the muscles, preparing us to confront or escape danger. The hypothalamus stimulates the release of adrenaline (epinephrine)[3] from the center of the adrenal gland. Another hormone from the hypothalamus sends a message to the nearby pituitary gland, instructing it to send yet another message to the outside part of the adrenal gland, adjacent to the kidney. The adrenal gland releases cortisol and similar hormones called glucocorticoids(1).

Each part of this cascade has important functions designed to get you out of trouble. The sympathetic nervous system response primes for fight or flight through direct nerve stimulation and by releasing epinephrine into your blood stream. Your muscles are prepared for you to confront the stressor.

Cortisol makes the process more efficient by shutting down unneeded body functions. It shuts off digestion. Cortisol shuts down body repair and immunity. Fending off an infection can be delayed. The pancreas is stimulated to release glucagon, which releases energy into the bloodstream by prompting the liver to break down stores of glycogen into glucose, quickly feeding muscles. Prolactin is secreted to shut down reproduction and other activities that don't provide an immediate life-saving effect. This description oversimplifies the immensely detailed process, but for our purposes the sympathetic nervous system, as well as release of epinephrine and cortisol, produces the response to stress.

There are important gender differences when describing the stress response. The hormone oxytocin is secreted during an acute stress response. Oxytocin also acts as a neurotransmitter and has a variety of other effects, including stimulating the uterus to contract and enabling lactating breasts to let-down milk. Oxytocin also increases social support and is involved in trust(8). It's the 'tend and befriend' hormone. Women may respond differently to an acute stressor because their brains produce a higher level of oxytocin in acutely stressful situations. When a man, woman and their child are faced with a threat, the man may fight or flee, while the woman would likely tend to her child. A group of women may work together to face a threat. The distinction may not seem so stark, but elements of it are present in the stress responses we'll be discussing and may account for gender differences in a range of behaviors.

The stress system was designed to address a threat that required a quick response. But it can't stay primed for too long. Once the threat is resolved, the body enters a recovery phase. Your fast breathing and rapid heartbeat subside, and you take a well-deserved rest. If you didn't survive, you took your final rest. Epinephrine and cortisol are no longer secreted, and the remaining hormones circulating in your bloodstream are metabolized. Recurring threats reawaken the sympathetic nervous system's stress response. These responses to stress had an evolutionary purpose: to help you survive(1, 9).

How to measure the stress response? One is to assay levels of circulating hormones. These can be detected in blood and urine samples. But these methods, drawing blood or collecting urine, can be stressful themselves. Saliva is more easily and less stressfully collected; the patient simply spits on a piece of absorbent paper. Cortisol is typically measured this way. Cortisol levels fluctuate during the day in a typical pattern, so experimentally it usually needs to be collected first thing in the morning.

Cortisol is deposited in the growing hair shaft, and hair grows about a centimeter (a third of an inch) each month. Taking hair samples and cutting them into pieces for cortisol assay is a useful test to gauge how much stress someone has been under over a longer period of time than a single day.

Hair cortisol levels in people with chronic pain show higher levels than those not in pain(10). Non-minority subjects of higher socioeconomic status have lower hair cortisol and lower perceived stress(11). This was not found for minorities. Many research studies now demonstrate higher hair cortisol, for example, in lower SES preschoolers, those with major depression, the unemployed, teachers with considerable effort–reward imbalance, and those doing shift work(12–14).

Other surrogate markers include measuring blood pressure, cardiac reactivity, blood clotting ability related to fibrinogen levels in the blood, cognitive function and a whole host of others. There is no single parameter to measure how much stress you are under at a particular time. Consider how stress varies throughout our lives.

Stress Throughout the Life Course

Stress in early life is a vital part of becoming a well-adapted adult. An infant who is challenged to stand upright without support experiences positive stress, which is a moderate, short-lived response that enables learning how to stand and walk. Such positive stress, and learning to adjust to it, is healthy development. The child learns to control and manage stress with the support of generally safe, warm, and positive relationships with caring adults. A child meeting new people, dealing with frustration, or overcoming a fear of animals can experience a positive stress response. This is normal. Such stress is short lived, accompanied by brief increases in stress hormones and rapid recovery to baseline status.

This positive stress helps the young brain develop as it makes and remakes various neural connections. The visual aspects of the brain are especially active in the early months after birth, followed by engaging hearing pathways. Sight and sound stimuli are vital for early brain development. After a year or two, the frontal cortex—the social part of our brain—is making and remaking neural connections. For this we need interaction with others, typically other children. Isolation wreaks psychological havoc on orphans who are denied human touch and interaction, as seen with the Romanian orphans we discussed in Chapter 5, as well as neglected infants and children.

Tolerable stress is generally brief and involves a situation that could harm the child, but the presence of supportive adults helps the body recover from potentially damaging events. Protective adult relationships help the child adapt. Examples of stressful events include the death or serious illness of a loved one, a frightening accident, or parental separation. In the absence of supportive relationships, such stress becomes toxic.

Toxic stress refers to strong, frequent, uncontrolled and prolonged activation of the stress response without attendant support from caring adults(15). Having more adverse childhood experiences—a higher ACE score—transforms tolerable stress into toxic stress. Being raised in an environment with emotional or physical abuse, being neglected, or being part of a dysfunctional family exposes the growing child to toxic stress, especially without adequate adult support.

Poverty in infancy is a type of toxic stress for which there is no cure later in life. As these infants age, they show more signs of elevated cortisol levels than those from richer families. Brain development is compromised, causing later impairments in learning, behavior and health. Effects of toxic stress in early life lead to a weaker immune system and higher levels of inflammatory markers that portend worse health as the child ages. Three or more ACEs result in steeper increases in hair cortisol with aging.

There are myriad early life stressors that can be studied in experimental situations. Consider getting infected with the common cold. The Pittsburgh Common Cold Studies, headed by Dr. Sheldon Cohen, took healthy volunteers and inoculated them with the cold virus, then measured the illness outcomes by the weight of tissues they used to blow nasal secretions. They looked at various measures of socioeconomic status for the volunteers including whether they owned their own home and whether their parents owned their own home for each childhood year. Those adults who own their own homes got fewer and less severe colds. How long their parents owned their homes while they were children was associated with developing less severe colds. An adult's immune system reflects stress in early life including whether that person's parents owned their own home. Again, poorer people, or those with poorer parents, have poorer health(16).

The stress that a pregnant woman experiences may have significant health effects on the fetus, and eventually the adult that infant becomes. The evidence from the Dutch Hunger Winter in Chapter 5 demonstrated that nutritional stress on the fetus can have lifelong effects, even spilling over into the next generation. Other forms of stress have impacts on the fetal programming of adult disease model described earlier. Psychological stress during pregnancy can lead to a higher risk of the infant being born prematurely, of low birthweight or even stillborn. Such stress impacts later health. Hair cortisol levels in women who deliver prematurely are related to their newborns' gestational age(17). The more stress a pregnant woman suffers, the more likely she is to have a premature baby, and such risk is greater among African Americans in the United States.

One series of studies compared the outcomes of healthy women in their 20s born to women who did and did not experience significant stress in their pregnancies. Stress during pregnancy was categorized as one of our major life events, comparable to the death of a close family member, serious illness of someone close, severe financial problems, relationship conflicts such as breakup or paternity denial, or becoming a political refugee. These are serious stressors, not just a bad hair day. Mothers who had more such psychosocial stressors while pregnant produced children who, upon reaching adulthood in their 20s, displayed a variety of abnormal physiological parameters that placed them at increased risk of chronic diseases as they aged(18).

Stress before conceiving, pre-conception stress, is also related to the probability of having a low birthweight baby. This association has been demonstrated through hair cortisol and self-reports in studies in the United States and elsewhere where racialized inequities are seen(19).

'Allostatic load' refers to the cumulative stress-induced burden on the body resulting from responses to repeated stressors and coping attempts. Consider it stress's long-term wear and tear(20). Frequent stress and the inability to turn off the stressor results in elevated blood pressure which increases the risk for heart attacks or myocardial infarctions. One study of men admitted to a hospital with a heart attack had collected samples of hair over the preceding three months and were compared to those admitted to an internal medicine service without this or a stroke diagnosis(21). The results showed that rising cortisol levels over the three months, demonstrating cumulative chronic stress, was associated with the infarction. Continued stress can increase the ability of the blood to clot and also lead to an elevated chance of heart attack and stroke.

Higher allostatic load is also seen people where COVID-19 has raged, especially among healthcare and essential workers.

If one aspect of the stress response, say cortisol secretion, is inadequate to deal with the threat, other mechanisms may step in and decrease or increase immune function. Some people have compromised immunity, while others have a hyperactive system and face so-called auto-immune diseases. There the stress response produces antibodies that target the body's own tissues as threats. This can lead to diseases such as rheumatoid arthritis (where antibodies attack joints) and lupus (where organs such as lungs and kidneys are assaulted). People with auto-immune diseases are more likely to have a significant SARS-CoV-2 infection. The opposite also occurs, namely, getting COVID-19 can trigger an auto-immune response, termed a cytokine storm, where the immune system overreacts, and the body attacks the lungs resulting in more severe infection complications.

With repeated activation, the stress response may weaken, so that when the big challenge comes, the immune system may not be able to respond adequately. Those who may have an attenuated cortisol response to stress include people with symptomatic HIV infection, women with metastatic breast cancer, children with high ACE scores, burned-out high school teachers and frontline workers during the COVID-19 pandemic.

Allostatic load can be measured using a variety of body parameters including blood pressure, cholesterol, weight, and how well your body handles glucose(22). Allostatic load increases with age. African Americans have higher levels of allostatic load than Whites, and poorer people also demonstrate more load. The process of weathering discussed in the last chapter also affects Blacks more.

"Shit Life Syndrome" describes many peoples' lives, in which they do meaningless work and struggle to maintain some semblance of dignity, yet are prey to an early death. Deaths of despair were mentioned in Chapter 3. Our declining health in the United States can be considered the result of the dehumanizing processes, like mouse work, taking place in our society. Life often fails to work out as well as expected. Stress and high allostatic load are the resulting processes, leading to worse health. This syndrome is not limited to the poor; it touches everyone, including the rich.

Post-traumatic stress disorder, or PTSD, is the condition in which a previous traumatic event—an extreme acute stressor or repeated series of stressful events—continues to affect that person long after the traumatic event is over. The trigger typically involves interpersonal violence. Victims may experience flashbacks of the event and hyperarousal or avoidance of reminders of the provoking event. In such people, the allostatic load can be so high that given another severe stressor, the individual can't mount a normal stress response. There is considerable stimulation of the pituitary to release cortisol, but release of the hormone is impaired. Cortisol levels may be low, and the daily variation absent. Such PTSD stress has shrunk the hippocampus and compromised other parts of the brain responsible for activating the stress effect(23). PTSD among military veterans is increasing in the USA as a result of the many unsuccessful wars the country has engaged in. Other conditions which commonly produce PTSD in our society include rape, childhood abuse, and physical assault.

Being raised as a child in low socioeconomic circumstances portend greater risk as an adult in acquiring COVID-19. Among U.S. counties, those with higher socioeconomic status had lower exposure to the virus and better outcomes(24). This effect likely began in early life and is another example of how inequality kills.

Biological Mechanisms Underlying Stress

Biological mechanisms which underlie stress that later link with disease consider inflammation as the primary process associated with adult chronic diseases. I learned in medical school that inflammation was the body's short-term response to fighting harmful stimuli by, for example, isolating an infection inside an abscess. Besides helping such an acute threat, the cells responsible for inflammation are found in many chronic disease conditions. A host of common diseases, including atherosclerosis (narrowing of the arteries supplying heart muscle), allergies, HIV, AIDS and COVID-19 are considered inflammatory disorders.

Higher levels of markers of inflammation portend worse health outcomes. Pathways linking inflammation with the immune system and social adversity in early life—poverty, low education, being raised by a single mother, etc.— increase allostatic load and lead to chronic illness. Many studies show that those of lower SES have more signs of inflammation. Production of C-Reactive Protein (CRP), an increasingly common blood test, is stimulated by higher levels of inflammatory cells. Sustained higher levels of CRP are associated with having a heart attack or stroke. CRP values increase among those of lower SES, and in those with less education(25). Levels of CRP appear to predict the severity and progression of COVID-19, in hospitalized patients. The gradient between SES and inflammatory markers varies by race or ethnicity. Levels are higher in Black people than in White people; even wealthy Black people have significantly higher levels when compared to wealthy Whites(26). Once again, poorer people can expect to have poorer health in addition to suffering the direct impacts of racism for people of color.

Serious COVID-19 often presents with hyperactive inflammation, the cytokine storm mentioned earlier. Cytokines are specific cells carrying out the inflammatory response. When they invade the lungs of someone infected with COVID-19, they cause severe respiratory distress requiring ventilatory support.

One disturbing example of the socioeconomic status health gradient looks at outcomes for young children who receive heart transplants. Overall, in the United States, those children who are of lower socioeconomic status are more likely to have worse outcomes and reject transplanted hearts(27). These lower SES children have not yet engaged in behaviors that might harm their health and lead to rejection, which means that stress of being lower status alone may account for the higher rate of rejection. Varying access to healthcare does not explain the difference, because elsewhere, in countries with universal health-care systems, the same result is found in child heart transplants. Being born poor or falling into financial trouble is bad for your health regardless of your individual efforts to be healthy.

Poorer people have poorer functioning organs. Ask a healthcare practitioner who has been working in diverse practice situations over a long period of time if they have observed poorer patients getting sicker. One suggested reason for why various medical care training curriculums avoid drawing attention to the effects of lower socioeconomic status on organs and health is that treatments for poverty or low socioeconomic status are not considered a subject for study in school. Similarly, some reason that why bring up ACEs in adults if we have no standardized treatments for conditions occurring long ago?

Consider organ function of the lung which can be measured with a simple test that is easily administered without much stress. To test your lungs, take a breath and exhale as much as you can. Then take the deepest breath you are capable of and blow it out as fast as you can. The volume of air you blow out in one second is called the "Forced Expiratory Volume 1," or FEV_1. Being able to blow out more air in one second indicates healthier lungs. Consistent with our previous findings, adults and children from richer or more educated families tend to have better functioning lungs. This difference is found around the world(28). The gradient remains after adjusting for cigarette smoking, and various occupational exposures which may harm the lungs, as well as racial categories. It is unlikely there is a single organ in the human body for which this isn't true. Hearts, kidneys, brains, gastrointestinal systems, reproductive organs and others are more difficult to study, because invasive procedures, such as drawing blood or inserting a catheter, are required to observe them, but when these studies are done the same result is found. Poorer people have poorer functioning organs.

Why the gradient in lung function? Early life is when SES matters most for lung health. Lower birth weight means that there was some type of compromise during the fetal period when lungs were being developed. Lower birth weights are more common in poorer people. Lower weight gain in childhood also leads to poorer functioning adult lungs. Taking lung function as an example, we can explore how early life can influence how well body organs work.

Epigenetics demonstrates how our environment gets under our skin. Poorer children are exposed to various physical, social, and economic conditions that damage their health, not necessarily through any health-related behavioral fault of their own. The idea that nurture complements nature (your genes) and that nurture can be passed to future generations is a very old concept that now has scientific validation.

Epigenetics means above or beyond genetics, and studies heritable ways in how genes are expressed. It explains how the environment affects the expression of genetic material. Genes can be silent or loud. Does the gene shout or whisper? The social, economic and physical environment can be seen as changing the way genes are expressed. These changes can be passed from one generation to the next without changing the actual genes. Epigenetic changes can be self-perpetuating or reversible.

In biology, or introductory biochemistry, you likely learned that genes are made up of strands of DNA inside our cells that code for a process of protein production. The resulting proteins enable your body to carry out many vital functions. These proteins are made in the body, as opposed to proteins we ingest as food. Epigenetic modifications of the gene result from several mechanisms, including adding methyl groups (methylation being the most studied so far) that change gene expression. Another epigenetic process is histone modification, which can affect a great amount of genetic expression in a similar manner. The genes themselves don't change; how they are expressed differs. To better understand them, consider how punctuation changes the meaning of a sentence:

- A woman without her man is nothing.
- A woman, without her, man is nothing.
- The words are the same, but how we punctuate the sentence can convey opposite meanings.

These "punctuation marks" are sensitive to environmental signals. They allow our bodies to adapt to the fast-paced and ever-changing world we live in.

Our lung function results stem from early life DNA methylation and histone modifications that change the structure of the lung, making for either better or worse breathing as the infant grows and develops into an adult. Being compromised in early life, as evidenced by lower birth weight and poor child weight gain—more common among individuals of lower SES—forever affects lung (and other organ) function. The higher prevalence of asthma among poorer children and those living in deprived areas is a powerful example of the impact of inequality on lung function and disease.

A number of experiments on animals help us to better understand the impacts of environmental stress on the body. Studies of rats and how rat mothers raise their pups demonstrate contrasting behaviors regarding mothering and attentive parenting. Experimental studies were carried out by Michael Meaney's group in Montreal beginning in the 1980s that built upon earlier work where rat pups who were separated from their mothers for brief periods in early life were found to have decreased stress responses as adults as well as other adverse health outcomes.

Meaney's group found some rat mothers engaged in considerable licking and grooming of the baby rats while others did not. Consider licking and grooming as effective parenting. Being licked and groomed in early life leads to healthier adult rats. Take two groups of rat mothers, one group licks and grooms their pups and another group that does not. Female rat pups of licking and grooming mothers tend to lick and groom their pups when mature, while those from non-licking and grooming mothers do not. This trait seems to be genetic. In cross-fostering experiments where pups from licking and grooming mothers are transferred immediately after birth to non-licking and grooming mothers, and vice versa, they found that whether a pup was licked or groomed determined the behavior it engaged in when it became a mother. The behavior is passed on to the next generation not by changing the genetic structure in any way, but rather through epigenetic mechanisms. The researchers figured out the specific epigenetic processes for the rat pups who were licked and groomed. They ended up being less stressed as they got older and healthier(29). Good mothering (and parenting in general) in early life leads to better health by inhibiting stress-induced aging. Children inherit their parents' genes as well as their parenting environments, impacting how they develop and their resulting health as adults.

Epigenetics is a nascent field with much to be learned. What matters most is understanding that nurture, in other words your environment—physical, social, emotional, economic—begins affecting you even before you're born. And it ultimately has profound effects on your health throughout life. Nature, your genetic make-up, also matters of course.

One more aspect of genetics and gene expression affects your health: telomeres. Telomeres, a vital part of biology, could be the single encompassing mechanism that explains how poverty affects your lifelong health. Can the fountain of youth spring from telomeres to become our holy grail?

Chromosomes are where your genes reside. We each have 23 pairs in all our cells. Telomeres are the complexes at the end of chromosomes, which protect DNA from unraveling. Think of them as the plastic or metal caps on the end of shoelaces that perform the same mechanical function. If they fall off or break, it becomes more difficult to thread the shoelaces into the holes. As your cells divide, these chromosomal caps shorten slightly. If they get too short, the cell dies. Telomeres were first hypothesized in the 1930s, but further details were not worked out until the 1970s. An enzyme telomerase, produced in the body, lengthens or repairs telomeres.

Telomeres naturally shorten with age. But they can also shorten in early life if the child is raised in a stressful environment. More adversity in early life such as exposure to domestic violence and bullying along with more child maltreatment results in shorter telomeres(30). The mother's stress levels during pregnancy can also affect the telomere length of her child(31). Telomeres shorten with more chronic stress. A study with disadvantaged African American children in New Orleans showed that neighborhood poverty levels were associated with shorter telomeres(32). Discrimination in older Black people is also associated with shorter telomeres. Geronimus, who developed weathering in the previous chapter, estimates Black women, aged 49–55, are 7.5 years older than White women on account of shorter telomeres(33). Consider telomere length as a biological marker of your age, distinct from your chronological age, that is, telomere age is typically different from your age in years.

Elizabeth Blackburn, who won a Nobel Prize for her telomere work, writes, "From the first moments of life, telomeres may be a measure of social and health inequalities." Other studies suggest the degree of telomere shortening predicts mortality, although in some populations this is reversed at very old ages(34). Again, like so many population-level measures considered in this book, your telomere length is not your destiny. The concept merely reflects population averages. There will always be exceptions.

There will also always be variation, which leads us to ask, what about comparisons of stress and health outcomes across countries?

Cross-National Stress Responses

Stress impacts biology and poor people are more likely to live with higher levels of stress than wealthier people, a correlation observed on a variety of levels. Looking on the cellular level at DNA, we see this correlation in the form of epigenetics, telomeres, and inflammatory markers. When it comes to cells grouped into organs, we've seen that poorer people have poorer functioning organs. We have seen that poverty leaves its mark in the form of overall worse health. One cross-national study observing the stress response was carried out in the 1990s and compared Linkoping in Sweden with nearby Vilnius in Lithuania. They found that heart disease mortality rates of middle-aged men were four times higher in Lithuania than in Sweden. There were only small differences among the cities in the traditional risk factors considered such as blood pressure, cholesterol, and smoking. There was higher job strain and lower social support in the Lithuanian men compared to Swedes resulting from the stress of the Soviet Union collapse in 1991. World War II affected Lithuania more than Sweden so early life factors were likely at work. The study took 50-year-old men in both cities and subjected them to a standardized laboratory stress test (anger recall, mental arithmetic, and hand immersion in ice water). They measured the cortisol and cardiovascular response, namely, what the baseline levels were and how they adjusted to stress. The subjects were then told to relax. As expected, heart rates and blood pressure rose in both groups when exposed to the laboratory stressors without much difference between them. Baseline cortisol was higher in the Vilnius men, but did not rise as much as in those from Linkoping. This finding is consistent with men in Vilnius being burned out and not being able to mount as effective a response when stressed, and their having a higher risk of heart attacks(35). Those with lower socioeconomic status in both cities had worse outcomes.

Similar mechanisms are found in various forms of burnout common in advanced societies today. Burnout, a term coined in 1974, is a state of emotional, physical and mental exhaustion caused by excessive and prolonged stress. There are many existing studies of burnout in surgical trainees with different countries exhibiting different rates likely because of the different stresses they are subject to. COVID-19 produced considerable burnout among many other healthcare workers caring for such patients. Burnout and compassion fatigue are hot topics as pandemic exhaustion has set in.

Coping with Stress

In response to our rising stress, a global industry has emerged to help us cope with this phenomenon. We are offered medications (and illicit drugs) to alleviate our anxieties, alcohol to calm our nerves, crystals and amulets, meditations and psychotherapy, calming lights, aroma therapy, candles and oils, massages and relaxation tanks, even expensive support pets ostensibly trained to calm us. There are many products and services we can now purchase to ease our stress.

Yet many of the coping mechanisms people adopt to deal with chronic stress can be bad for health. Consider the high intake of sugar in modern diets. Sugar consumption has increased thirty-fold in the United States over the last 150 years. Sugar is added to many processed foods that are tasty and convenient to prepare. Part of the stress response requires mobilization of body energy stores to respond to the threat. Consuming energy in the form of sugar makes this process more efficient and does not deplete body energy stores. Sugar-sweetened beverages are the largest sources of added sugars in the diets of American children and adults, which can lead to diabetes and obesity. It also shortens telomeres.

Yet so-called "comfort foods," containing sugar and fat, also help people experience less stress by inhibiting cortisol secretion, decreasing stress reactivity and prompting the release of endorphins in the brain(36). Poorer people are more likely to overeat or have other dysfunctional eating patterns, as such stress-relieving foods become addictive. The next chapter will explore diets in greater detail.

Other stress coping mechanisms include smoking cigarettes. Smoking today in the United States is mostly done by poorer people and exists as a coping mechanism which helps them face the endless stress of their daily lives.

The debate is still on as to whether some alcohol use is beneficial, but there is much alcohol abuse that wrecks many lives. We have discussed opioid use before. This country has the highest opioid use per person of any nation, consistent with our high levels of experienced stress compared with other nations.

Ultimately, however, decreasing poverty and economic inequality will have far more beneficial effects on reducing the population levels of stress in our society than the plethora of stress-reducing products and services increasingly promoted in the media and online.

Conclusion

We have considered that economic inequality, the stress of living among varying degrees of plenty, is written into our cells, our organs, ourselves as individuals, and expressed outwardly to our communities and entire countries. Being richer within a society is associated with healthier biology, though richer countries are not necessarily healthier than poorer ones, as the United States, the richest nation in world history, but far from the healthiest, demonstrates. This chapter helps us to further understand how inequality and suboptimal conditions in early life impact our biology and causes worse health.

We must consider the political choices we have made to have these outcomes. To do so, the next chapter will present another look at our components, cells, organs, individuals and populations and consider how social systems change— and what needs to be done to make that happen.

Questions to Consider and Discuss

1. Given the economic opportunities for having a great deal of stress in a community, what can be done to fundamentally de-stress society?
2. How do you cope with stress individually? What changes might you make after understanding this chapter?

Notes

1. Selye was an expert witness for the tobacco industry and defended their interests, details of which were only published in 2011.
2. These health impacts included infectious agents that spread from animals to humans as we domesticated animals and lived closer to wild habitats. Cross-species transmission has continued to pose threats, with Lyme disease coming from deer ticks associated with

expanding housing into wooded, rural areas, while HIV/AIDS originated in monkeys and SARS-CoV-2 is thought to come to humans from bats.

3. Epinephrine and adrenaline mean the same substance. Adrenalin® is a patented drug in the United States.

References

1. Sapolsky RM. Why Zebras Don't Get Ulcers: The Acclaimed Guide to Stress, Stress-Related Diseases and Coping. 3rd edition. New York, NY: Henry Holt; 2004.

2. Sapolsky RM. The Health-Wealth Gap. Scientific American. November, 2018, pp. 62–7.

3. Ray J. Americans' Stress, Worry and Anger Intensified in 2018 Washington, D.C.: Gallup; 2019 [cited 2019 April 25]. Available from: https://news.gallup.com/poll/249098/americans-stress-worry-anger-intensified-2018.aspx?utm_source=link_wwwv9&utm_campaign=item_248900&utm_medium=copy.

4. Hanson PG. The Joy of Stress. Kansas City: Andrews, McMeel & Parker; 1986.

5. Marcus-Newhall A, Pedersen WC, Carlson M, Miller N. Displaced Aggression Is Alive and Well: A Meta-Analytic Review. Journal of Personality and Social Psychology. 2000; 78(4):670–89.

6. Scheff TJ. Shame and Conformity: The Deference-Emotion System. American Sociological Review. 1988;53(3):395–406.

7. American Psychological Association. Stress in America 2020 A National Mental Health Crisis. Washington, D.C.: American Psychological Association; 2020.

8. Zak PJ. The Moral Molecule: the Source of Love and Prosperity. New York, NY: Dutton; 2012.

9. Sapolsky RM. Behave: The Biology of Humans at Our Best and Worst. New York, NY: Penguin; 2017.

10. Van Uum SHM, Sauvé B, Fraser LA, Morley-Forster P, Paul TL, Koren G. Elevated Content of Cortisol in Hair of Patients With Severe Chronic Pain: A Novel Biomarker for Stress. Stress: The International Journal on the Biology of Stress. 2008;11(6): 483–8.

11. O'Brien KM, Tronick EZ, Moore CL. Relationship between Hair Cortisol and Perceived Chronic Stress in a Diverse Sample. Stress and Health. 2013;29(4):337–44.

12. Groeneveld MG, Vermeer HJ, Linting M, Noppe G, van Rossum EFC, van Ijzendoorn MH. Children's Hair Cortisol as a Biomarker of Stress at School Entry. Stress: The International Journal on the Biology of Stress. 2013;16(6):711–5.

13. Manenschijn L, van Kruysbergen R, de Jong FH, Koper JW, van Rossum EFC. Shift Work at Young Age Is Associated With Elevated Long-Term Cortisol Levels and Body Mass Index. Journal of Clinical Endocrinology & Metabolism. 2011;96(11):E1862–E5.

14. Qi XL, Zhang J, Liu YP, Ji S, Chen Z, Sluiter JK, et al. Relationship between Effort-Reward Imbalance and Hair Cortisol Concentration in Female Kindergarten Teachers. Journal of Psychosomatic Research. 2014;76(4):329–32.

15. Shonkoff JP, Slopen N, Williams DR. Early Childhood Adversity, Toxic Stress, and the Impacts of Racism on the Foundations of Health. Annual Review of Public Health. 2021;42(1):115–34.

16. Cohen S, Doyle WJ, Turner RB, Alper CM, Skoner DP. Childhood Socioeconomic Status and Host Resistance to Infectious Illness in Adulthood. Psychosom Med. 2004; 66(4):553–8.

17. Kramer MS, Lydon J, Seguin L, Goulet L, Kahn SR, McNamara H, et al. Stress Pathways to Spontaneous Preterm Birth: The Role of Stressors, Psychological Distress, and Stress Hormones. American Journal of Epidemiology. 2009;169(11):1319–26.

18. Entringer S, Kumsta R, Nelson EL, Hellhammer DH, Wadhwa PD, Wust S. Influence of Prenatal Psychosocial Stress on Cytokine Production in Adult Women. Developmental Psychobiology. 2008;50(6):579–87.

19. Strutz KL, Hogan VK, Siega-Riz AM, Suchindran CM, Halpern CT, Hussey JM. Preconception Stress, Birth Weight, and Birth Weight Disparities Among US Women. American Journal of Public Health. 2014;104(8):e125–e32.

20. McEwen BS. Protective and Damaging Effects of Stress Mediators. New England Journal of Medicine. 1998;338(3):171–9.

21. Pereg D, Gow R, Mosseri M, Lishner M, Rieder M, Van Uum S, et al. Hair Cortisol and the Risk for Acute Myocardial Infarction in Adult Men. Stress-the International Journal on the Biology of Stress. 2011;14(1):73–81.

22. Geronimus AT, Hicken M, Keene D, Bound J. "Weathering" and Age Patterns of Allostatic Load Scores Among Blacks and Whites in the United States. American Journal of Public Health. 2006;96(5):826–33.

23. McEwen BS. Allostasis and Allostatic Load: Implications for Neuropsychopharmacology. Neuropsychopharmacology. 2000;22(2):108–24.

24. Clouston SAP, Natale G, Link BG. Socioeconomic Inequalities in the Spread of Coronavirus-19 in the United States: A Examination of the Emergence of Social Inequalities. Social Science & Medicine. 2021;268:113554.

25. Vineis P, Delpierre C, Castagné R, Fiorito G, McCrory C, Kivimaki M, et al. Health Inequalities: Embodied Evidence Across Biological Layers. Social Science & Medicine. 2020;246:112781.

26. Ranjit N, Diez-Roux AV, Shea S, Cushman M, Ni H, Seeman T. Socioeconomic Position, Race/Ethnicity, and Inflammation in the Multi-Ethnic Study of Atherosclerosis. Circulation. 2007;116(21):2383–90.

27. Singh TP, Blume ED, Naftel DC, Foushee MT, Kirklin JK, Addonizio L, et al. Association of Race and Socioeconomic Position With Outcomes in Pediatric Heart Transplant Recipients. American Journal of Transplantation. 2010;10(9):2116–23.

28. Hegewald MJ, Crapo RO. Socioeconomic Status and Lung Function. Chest. 2007;132(5):1608–14.

29. Bouvette-Turcot A-A, Meaney MJ, O'Donnell KJ. Epigenetics and Early Life Adversity: Current Evidence and Considerations for Epigenetic Studies in the Context of Child Maltreatment In: Noll JG, Shalev I, Noll JG, Shalev I, editors. The Biology of Early Life Stress: Understanding Child Maltreatment and Trauma. Cham, Switzerland: Springer; 2018. pp. 89–119.

30. Kiecolt-Glaser JK, Gouin JP, Weng NP, Malarkey WB, Beversdorf DQ, Glaser R. Childhood Adversity Heightens the Impact of Later-Life Caregiving Stress on Telomere Length and Inflammation. Psychosomatic Medicine. 2011;73(1):16–22.

31. Entringer S, Epel ES, Kumsta R, Lin J, Hellhammer DH, Blackburn EH, et al. Stress Exposure in Intrauterine Life Is Associated With Shorter Telomere Length in Young Adulthood. Proceedings of the National Academy of Sciences. 2011;108(33):E513–E8.

32. Theall KP, Brett ZH, Shirtcliff EA, Dunn EC, Drury SS. Neighborhood Disorder and Telomeres: Connecting Children's Exposure to Community Level Stress and Cellular Response. Social Science & Medicine. 2013;85(0):50–8.

33. Geronimus AT, Pearson JA, Linnenbringer E, Schulz AJ, Reyes AG, Epel ES, et al. Race-Ethnicity, Poverty, Urban Stressors, and Telomere Length in a Detroit Community-Based Sample. Journal of Health and Social Behavior. 2015;56(2):199–224.
34. Blackburn EH, Epel E. The Telomere Effect: A Revolutionary Approach to Living Younger, Healthier, Longer. New York, NY: Grand Central Publishing; 2017.
35. Kristenson M, Eriksen HR, Sluiter JK, Starke D, Ursin H. Psychobiological Mechanisms of Socioeconomic Differences in Health. Social Science & Medicine. 2004;58(8): 1511–22.
36. Tryon MS, DeCant R, Laugero KD. Having Your Cake and Eating It Too: A Habit of Comfort Food May Link Chronic Social Stress Exposure and Acute Stress-Induced Cortisol Hyporesponsiveness. Physiology & Behavior. 2013;114-115:32–7.

Chapter 8

Our Health Depends on Political Choices

> The primary determinants of disease are mainly economic and social, and therefore its remedies must also be economic and social. Medicine and politics cannot and should not be kept apart.
>
> *Geoffrey Rose(1)*

The upstream factors, root, or fundamental causes of health production center around economic and political systems as well as culture. Over the last half century, political policies at the U.S. state level, reflecting conservative and liberal orientations, have affected trends in health outcomes. We now turn to dissecting populations and their components to see how political choices impact health.

Cells, Organs, Individuals, Populations

Our bodies are just trillions of cells stuck together, and these cells are integrated into communities forming our organs. Your brain, heart, blood, kidneys, lungs, and pancreas are all specialized cellular systems. What do they need to be healthy? If a group of heart muscle cells are deprived of oxygen or glucose because of a clotted artery, they die and you have a heart attack. Similarly in the brain when you have a stroke. Besides the right quantities of oxygen and glucose, what a group of cells needs depends on the organ. How should we produce healthy organs?

For better health, we are told to eat right, exercise, don't smoke, see our doctor, use a condom, and so on. Unfortunately, none of those guidelines have meaning at the cellular level. You can't tell a cell to exercise; that is not what they can choose to do. Blood cells move through your circulatory system because your heart pumps them. Bone cells are fixed in place. Similarly, you can't tell your lung cells to not inhale smoke. That is the individual's responsibility rather than the cell's. The same goes for using a condom or eating right. If you keep yourself healthy following the individual precepts, you expect your organs, and their cellular components, to be healthy as well.

DOI: 10.4324/9781003315889-9

In Chapter 2, we saw that medical care treated cells and organs, not the person. If we could treat the individual, rather than their cells and organs, then we would ensure they have a safe place to recover and suffer less stress, adequate nutrition, affordable medicine, and a baseline income. Lacking these safety nets, however, by segregating medical care from human care, we are limited in our ability to heal individuals. Our focus on the health of the individual assumes the health advice provided to one person will work for an entire population. In the COVIDian era we saw this prescription writ large as we were told to mask up, physically distance, and get immunized—all sound advice, but without consideration for differences among people's risk.

Are there factors that produce health in populations beyond what individuals do? In other words, are there elements that affect populations that have no individual counterparts in the same way that individual health advice has no cellular equivalents?

We need to discover those population level factors and get them operating. Then what individual humans do to advance their health doesn't matter as much as we're led to believe. This could explain why Japan is the country with the longest life expectancy despite its large proportion of male smokers. The population health approach utilizes such thinking—find out what produces health in a population and then implement those factors to make those within that population healthy. It is comparable to advising individuals to do what is best for their health. If individuals eat right, exercise, etc. their cells and organs become healthy as a byproduct of the entire body's better health.

The British epidemiologist Geoffrey Rose distinguished between sick individuals and sick populations in a seminal 1985 paper. He looked not at why some individuals had hypertension or high blood pressure, but at why some populations had widespread hypertension and others did not. Some of the highest blood pressures among adults are found among African Americans in the United States, while some of the most consistently low blood pressures are found in Africans in Africa. What factors are producing such a distinct difference among populations so similar?

Medical students are taught to consider why a particular patient has severe hypertension. The patient not taking their blood pressure medicine is a common reason, or they are obese, have kidney disease, or other risk factors. But doctors should broaden their gaze to consider why there is so much hypertension in the United States, or why we die so much younger than people in other societies.

Unfortunately, we don't ask these broader social questions because poor health has become normalized here. Rose asked us to consider not only the causes in an individual with an illness, but why some populations have more of that illness than another. When biologist Sandra Steingraber was diagnosed with bladder cancer in her early 20s and remarked that it ran in her family, her physician told her it was genetic. But Steingraber was adopted. After recovering, she set out to explore what was happening in her rural mid-western farm community that might explain the elevated cancer risk, discovering a multitude of carcinogens in the toxic chemicals sprayed in the fields that entered the water supply(2).

Rose pointed out that prevention strategies in sick populations would be different than those for sick individuals(1). For individuals one needs a screening program to identify those at high risk, and then regimens to modify behaviors and otherwise treat them. This expensive strategy leads to the astronomical costs of U.S. medical care. It is not effective given the poor health status we have compared to other nations. A prevention program aimed at the population might work to change societal norms. Let's consider smoking as an example.

It is now illegal to smoke in restaurants, airplanes, and most public places, and tobacco can no longer be advertised on TV, billboards, or public transport. These bans led to plummeting smoking rates and one rarely smells cigarette smoke anymore—a stark contrast from the mid-20th century when children routinely grew up in clouds of cigarette smoke at home, and smokers routinely lit up in cars, restaurants, airplanes, and elevators. To compensate for the lost sales, tobacco companies have increased internet advertising and point-of-sale marketing to specific groups defined by race, ethnicity, and income, among others. The poor, trying to cope with high levels of stress associated with their poverty and low status, are now targeted online with discount coupons and free packs of major cigarette brands. In our pandemic era many smokers have increased their consumption (with big increases in electronic cigarettes which contain nicotine and harmful chemicals). Fewer smokers sought help to quit smoking in 2020. Given the increased stress and isolation in our homes, with nicotine being among the most addictive chemicals, our cigarette consumption has increased in the pandemic.

The question these issues raise is if we did shift to a focus from the individual to the population, how would we go about treating this population? It is difficult to mandate a prescription—as we've seen with COVID-19—or even implement a vaccine program at the population level. But there are some steps we can take.

Treating the Population to Improve Our Health

Treating a population's health is much more difficult than giving individual advice, especially in the United States. Let's begin with some ideas and examples.

Strategies for treating populations do not motivate the medical care profession nor their patients. Doctors are trained to diagnose and treat *individual* illness and injury. Population prevention doesn't produce grateful patients in doctors' offices. Recall my frustration at trying to get smokers to stop smoking. It just didn't work. Patients want quick fixes for their health, but they also resist governmental interference in their behaviors, as COVID-19 has demonstrated.

Europeans first encountered tobacco when they settled in America. By the turn of the 20th century, many people, even children, smoked cigarettes.

Everyone was exposed to cigarette smoke. The first reports linking smoking to lung cancer appeared in the 1920s, but tobacco companies (subsidized by the U.S. government) heavily promoted their products as healthy. The harm of cigarette smoking was finally brought to public attention in the 1950s and early 1960s, and the tobacco industry responded by introducing filtered cigarettes, suggesting they were less harmful. By the 1970s and 1980s, the harm from secondhand smoke was well established, and laws began to limit where people could smoke. While there was initially a great deal of resistance to these laws, with people offended if asked to smoke outside, it now seems normal to do so and smoking rates have declined substantially in rich countries. In response, the tobacco industry has shifted its advertising to poorer nations where they recognize that today's teenager is tomorrow's addicted smoker, so poor youth are targeted with sales of single cigarettes common for those who can't afford a full pack. Over 80% of global cigarette smoking now occurs in middle- and low-income countries. Despite the success in reducing our rate of smoking at the population level, the problem of nicotine addiction remains, and this lethal but legal industry still receives government subsidies. In 2020, the U.S. tobacco farmers received a hundred million dollars in government payments, to help them through the coronavirus pandemic.

Given what we know of how harmful smoking is, how can Japan limit the damage? Through a culture of social solidarity. Have you ever seen a lone Japanese tourist in the United States? Pre-pandemic, we repeatedly saw groups of Japanese tourists, whereas the lone American tourist was found everywhere. *Wa*, or social solidarity, is the Japanese term for the collective harmony of social networks, an essential aspect of Japanese culture. Japanese distinguish *honne*, one's true feelings, with *tatemae*, the face one wears in public(3). This distinction contrasts with the individualist attitude, our American social norm. Could our proclivity toward individualism and our increasing lack of strong social and kinship ties be a factor in our higher mortality rate?

Western culture is more individualistic and analytic-thinking than East Asian culture, which is more interdependent and holistic-thinking. We can see this difference in our respective means of food production. In East Asian cultures, rice cultivation dominates, requiring massive collective labor. A rice field requires the coordinated efforts of the whole village, as fields are laboriously terraced and irrigated, the rice stocks planted, weeded, and harvested by hand, then threshed and pounded to remove the hard husks. In contrast, growing wheat or corn, or herding animals, is a far more solitary activity, as well as far more competitive as farmers compete for the highest market share. Scholars also attribute higher rates of violence and cultures of honor to herding cultures where men individually compete for the best grazing areas and economic success.

East Asian countries where Confucian philosophy predominates also tend to have a more cooperative and long-term orientation.

This collectivist orientation in Asian cultures may partially explain why in East Asia, countries such as China, Japan, Korea, and Taiwan, initially had very few COVID-19 cases and deaths. Dealing with COVID-19 requires collective responses, rather than the individualistic response many in the United States have embraced as their "right" not to wear masks, socially distance, or vaccinate. If anything, our individualism is growing even greater in the United States, making it all the more difficult to meet the challenges of public health crises.

Another population intervention considers environmental pollution, especially water and air pollution and exposure to various chemicals. Strong efforts were made in the 1960s to develop regulatory mechanisms—including creating the Environmental Protection Agency (EPA)—to limit exposure to pollution. This happened during a period of considerably less inequality in America. But as inequality has increased, recent federal administrations have prioritized corporate rights, and the substantial health gains from regulating toxic exposures have been relaxed. Examples include reversing the ban on the pesticide chlorpyrifos (linked to brain damage in children), limiting enforcement of mercury emissions, and lifting bans on oil and natural gas extraction.

Consider also workplace safety. The Occupational Safety and Health Act (OSHA) was enacted over 50 years ago. OSHA was established to transform workplaces to reduce injuries, illnesses, and fatalities. Still the rate of occupational deaths in the United States is four times greater than in the United Kingdom(4). Yet the legislation that was helping reduce that high death rate was de-regulated in the Trump era. Workplaces no longer need to keep detailed records of shop floor injuries and illnesses. Limits have now been placed on mining inspections as well as on the rights to organize and join a union. Fewer workers are now protected from hazardous exposures. Since the pandemic, workplace regulations have been further neglected, especially for essential workers who must often work without proper protection from the virus.

As these examples show, although we know a great deal about how to treat a population the current global political system is diverted away from those concepts with an increasing individual focus.

Leaving the Risk Factory

Despite the advances we have made in health by addressing problems at the societal level, medical care continues to address health by treating individuals, typically using a risk factor approach (trying to avoid conditions that make individuals more susceptible to illness or injury) discussed in Chapter 5.

Risk factors have been the dominant narrative about individual health in the United States for decades. We are overwhelmed with too much information. We focus on diagnosing diseases. If you think you are healthy you haven't had enough tests yet! Just by the process of deciding what is a normal test result, by doing enough tests we will find something abnormal even though the person is healthy. This may lead to more tests and associated harm.

Consider individuals with the risk factor of so-called bad cholesterol (that attached to Low Density Lipoprotein or LDL) and their chances of having a heart attack. Studies show that those with higher LDL are at greater risk of having a heart attack. Medical care tries to lower bad cholesterol with drugs in the hopes of averting heart attacks. These drugs, statins, target the liver affecting enzymes in hepatocytes or liver cells. We saw in Chapter 2 how little statins do to prolong life. Again, medical care treats cells in the hopes of benefitting individuals, while failing to address why we have so much bad cholesterol in the first place.

There are non-drug means for increasing good cholesterol (that attached to High Density Lipoproteins or HDL) which we hear about all the time, including exercise, avoiding smoking, losing weight, reducing sugar intake, changing the fats in your diet, consuming fatty fish, and increasing fiber intake. This approach hopes to promote heart health by modifying individual behaviors. If we were successful in eradicating heart disease as a cause of death, however, we would still not be the healthiest nation.

We can easily end up with a list of close to a hundred risk factors to be wary of, leading individuals to feeling conflicted and confused. Addressing population issues may be less stressful and produce better results. But they are problematic to implement because of their political nature—many politicians brand any effort to address health at the societal level as a threat to individual freedoms, while many citizens accept such spin as a violation of their American rights.

Consider COVID-19. The villain is an unseen virus. Infection doesn't produce pockmarks on the skin or cripple the person as with polio. Many reason, let's just forget about it and carry on with life as usual, presuming we can't trust what the government is telling us about COVID. That distrust is not surprising. Individual agency in America partly stems from increasing inequality producing less trust in government institutions. One consequence is that the country is increasingly divided by political tribalism—a tribalism that has been marked by vastly different perceptions of risk to COVID, and very different responses to both prevention and treatment. Without a coherent national strategy, we will continue to be hampered to control this plague while pursuing individual rights to ignore the threat.

If we know what needs to be done at the individual level to improve our health, what then are the salutary social processes that enhance health at the population level? They must include political actions that support early life, such as those that give parents the time and resources needed to raise healthy children, the subject of Chapter 5. As we've also discussed extensively, they need to address economic inequality too. How much inequality is there in the United States?

Decline in Social Cohesion and Rise of Individualism

We saw in Chapter 3 in our discussion of inequality that the rich don't want to share their wealth, so they developed ways to keep it. Since they pay for all their exclusive services, they don't want to be taxed. The 2017 1.5 trillion dollar U.S. tax-cut legislation is a prime example. Yet most of the people in the country hardly whimpered as this happened. Why?

The neoliberal transformation of society since the 1970s produced a system that allows the rich and powerful to have nearly everything they want. In the 1960s, there was tremendous popular resistance, as evidenced by the opposition to our invasion of Vietnam, the Civil Rights movement, rioting in inner cities, the democracy trials in Chicago, the shut-down of major universities, and much more. Social movements, then physical rather than virtual, threatened those in power.

Discussing uprisings in the 1960s, the Trilateral Commission's 1975 report titled, *The Crisis of Democracy*, said there could even be too much democracy(5). Too many people were exercising their rights in the sixties! What was needed was a cooling off of this excess of democracy. *Business Week*, on October 12, 1974 stated, "It will be a hard pill for many Americans to swallow—the idea of doing with less so that business can have more …. Nothing that this nation, or any other nation, has done in modern economic history compares in difficulty with the selling job that must be done to make people accept the new reality."(6) What was the selling job?

Selling ideas to Americans for more than a century is a major industry. President Woodrow Wilson was re-elected President in 1916 on a peace without victory platform, meaning that the country was not going to enter World War I. He formed the Committee on Public Information (Creel Commission) to successfully convince Americans to go to war. Sigmund Freud's nephew, Edward Bernays, was a major force developing this activity. In his 1928 book, *Propaganda*, Bernays pointed out that the real ruling power in the country were those who manipulated the habits and opinions of the masses, an invisible government, and was the true ruling force of the country(7). Power is most effective when least observable. Most of us believe we exercise our free will in our actions and thoughts. Recognizing the limitations of our critical thinking and acting skills is a challenge we all face.

What followed the selling job resulted in not only the restoration of the richest one percent's wealth share to never before seen levels but also the marketing to us that our role was to be individual consumers who spend more despite having less to spend. As economic inequality increased, we shopped with a vengeance. Yet hourly wages remained stagnant, even though productivity (the amount produced per worker) rose. Instead of demanding higher wages we borrowed our salaries by taking on higher credit card debt and getting home equity loans that were beyond our means to repay. We focused on our own new-found "needs" rather than our communities. This consumption combined with lower wages and increased job insecurity led to the 2008–9 banking crisis. Then came the COVID-19 crash. We now work together even less than before and have become more isolated than we've ever been.

More trusting societies have a smaller income gap. Among 84 nations studied, lower trust has severely impacted COVID-19 deaths with many more deaths in less trusting societies(8).

Being more isolated we have become more fearful of others. Insecurity about our status leads to withdrawal from social engagement. Instead of face-to-face contact, we turn to social media. We are increasingly 'alone together.' The stress resulting from our status anxiety tempts us to use alcohol, other drugs, and comfort food as a temporary fix. Such behaviors have vastly increased during the pandemic.

Markers of our individualism can be seen in trends such as the rise of tattoos and various body adornment and modification to reflect our independence. Graffiti emerged from a subculture into mainstream pop culture as a form of personal expression with its various tags that represent singular signatures. The nonstop barrage of selfies posted online, daily updates posted on how we feel, what we ate, and how cute our pets are, and endless books and articles telling us we're fabulous, amazing, and deserve the best keep our focus on ourselves. Narcissism is entrenched and encouraged in modern society(9). The iGeneration is all about ME(10). Young people who have grown up with the internet, prefer to spend their time on their smartphones rather than hanging out with each other. Even when they're with each other, they're connecting with strangers on their devices. The job of creating individual desire by big business, of making people accept the new reality, has been very successful. This shift created the moral decay described in Chapter 4.

Consider this allegory to grasp what has happened in society. Imagine a chauffeur who drives a sleek limousine through the streets of a major American city, with a billionaire in the back seat. Out of the window, the billionaire spots a homeless woman and her two children huddling in the cold, sharing a loaf of bread. He orders the chauffeur to stop the car. When the limo comes to a halt, the chauffeur opens the passenger door for the billionaire. The billionaire then walks over to the mother and snatches the loaf from her. He slips back into the car, and they drive on, leaving behind a baffled group of sidewalk witnesses. For his part, the chauffeur feels qualms about what his master has done because, unlike his employer, he has recently known hard times himself. But he drives on nonetheless. Let's call this the chauffeur's dilemma. It is a parable for life in the USA today.

Absurd as it seems, we are actually witnessing this scene as you read it. Or more exactly, about half of us are in the role of the chauffeur, opening the door for the billionaire, and the other half are watching from the sidewalk, bewildered and dismayed. And doing nothing about it.

Something has been going on between the front and the back of the car—something in the way of a private moral deal between the billionaire and the chauffeur. It's a deal that has already left the world a lot meaner but solves an emotional problem for some people who, given the way their own lives are being squeezed, find themselves with less empathy left over for others outside their social circle. In other words, we find our lives increasingly stressed, fast paced, and difficult, and we no longer look out for others. We need to understand this empathy squeeze to grasp why so many Americans think and act like the billionaire's chauffeur when they are not, in fact, employed by him. These ideas, this deal, as I have pointed out have the most profound influence on our health, far more than anything we can accomplish by changing our diet, exercising, stopping smoking, and all the things you are told to do.

Political Strategies for Producing Population Health

Population health considers the major determinants of the health of populations. Public health broadcasts individual health advice to the public which has major limitations for improving health. Defining politics is a political act, variously defined as, "Politics is about who has the right to tell whom what to do"[1] or "Politics is the shadow cast over society by big business"[2] or "politics is an interaction among groups of investors who compete for control of the state."[3] Another is, "the activities associated with the governance of a country or other area, especially the debate or conflict among individuals or parties having or hoping to achieve power." There are important commonalities, however.

Politics is about power, who has it, and how is it used. Consider some events during this century reflected in power politics. A political act, the destruction of New York's World Trade Towers in 2001, led to another political act, namely, the United States invading Afghanistan and Iraq. These wars led to immense tragedies accompanied by huge profits (more than 7 trillion dollars) accruing to investors in mostly American military industries. The United States lost both wars. Since its founding in 1776 the country has not been at war for less than 20 years. Warring is a major American pastime with huge economic benefits to large U.S. corporate investors. The 2008–9 banking crisis resulted from political choices made in the 1990s to de-regulate banking. The large investors, the banks, were bailed out, and none of the criminals went to jail or were even indicted. Those who suffered most were of limited financial means. Yet instead of limiting the power of these wealthy banks, various austerity programs have been put in place to limit payouts to poorer families. The COVID-19 crisis brings all these issues out into the open with our billionaire bonanza of pandemic profiteering during which one billionaire is created every 17 hours. Such increases in inequality resulting from the imbalance of power are behind our absolute health decline.

Power distance within nations can be ranked. With a large power distance income and other inequalities are expected and desired. Educational policy focuses on universities rather than secondary schools. Less powerful people are dependent on those with more. James Baldwin noted that the powerless must do their own dirty work, namely, the essential risky jobs that put them in harm's way, while the powerful have it done for them. With greater power distance in the workplace there are more supervisory personnel and a bigger wage gap.

We have a dysfunctional political system in incredibly rich America. Despite being a democracy where power is supposedly shared, our health is at best that of a middle-income country. How does such a system change?

How do policies and laws happen in the United States? University of Michigan political scientist John W. Kingdon in his book, *Agendas, Alternatives, and Public Policies*, considered policy changes in America(11). The original studies in the 1970s looked at health (care) maintenance organizations, national health (care) insurance, and deregulation of aviation, along with trucking, railroad, and waterway user charges. A later edition examined the Tax Reform Act, the Clinton Health Care Initiative, and the resulting federal budget changes of the Reagan revolution.

By studying how U.S. policies came into being over the last century, Kingdon concluded that three key concepts were required to push through new legislation. First, the problem must attract nationwide attention. Agenda setting. Kingdon's phrase, "An idea's time has come," is the unique window of opportunity during which a hot issue can lead to groundbreaking change. Windows of opportunity (also called the Overton Window after Joseph Overton, Vice President of the Mackinac Center for Public Policy) span a range of political possibilities for solutions(12). What determines when an idea's time has come in the United States remains a mystery. Almost a hundred years after the abolition of slavery, the Civil Rights Movement suddenly took hold and led to sweeping changes, though racism remains in many forms. The entire movement began as an idea at the local level, which eventually became national. After George Floyd's murder in 2020, the movement became global.

A second necessary component requires defining specific policy solutions. This work is often done by invisible players: civil servants, lobbyists, academics, specialist journalists, and legislative staff. Kingdon calls this alternative-specification. While these two processes—agenda setting and alternative-specification—are all that is necessary in other countries, such as the United Kingdom, they aren't enough in the United States.

Kingdon distinguishes three process streams: policy, politics, and problem. Our problem, American declining health status, isn't part of anyone's political or policy agenda at this point as there is almost no awareness of the problem at any level. It is not considered by the CDC Division of the Federal Department of Health and Human Services (DHHS) or DHHS itself. The CDC is primarily concerned with diseases. A former student of mine joined the CDC as an epidemic intelligence services officer. He details how the agency is focused specifically on high-profile diseases such as HIV, suicide, overdose, and COVID. Yet we remain indifferent to our declining national health.

We need to overcome this disregard, and have alternative-specification, or potential solutions, to the problem. The required policy, Kingdon argues, may be in a 'garbage can,' that is, a variety of diverse interests, objectives, and ideas often get dumped into a single legislative decision. There are often no obvious connections among the diverse and dissimilar contents of the 'garbage can.'

Recognition is not enough to bring about change. In the United States there needs to be a third component, a window of opportunity, for change to happen. The transforming events necessary to set the wheels in motion are not under control of the political process. They can take the form of a natural disaster, an economic depression, a war, or a major electoral realignment.

We've seen several such windows of opportunity, or transforming events, in this century. The terrorist attacks on September 11, 2001 quickly led to the passage of the Patriot Act, with all its enhanced surveillance mechanisms. The country's leaders had their eyes set on this legislation, with various drafts, years before the attacks occurred. This event led to two more wars which cost so many lives (at least a million, mostly citizens, of those two nations), but the small numbers (over 7,000) of American deaths are all we hear about. There were huge corporate profits from these wars. Hurricane Katrina could have been another, but little came of it politically. Today COVID-19 can provide this opportunity.

During the previous century, in the 1930s, the Great Depression was the window of opportunity that led to the New Deal and Social Security, as well as increased taxes on the rich. Details will be found in Chapter 9. The Russian launch of Sputnik in 1957 drove the United States to focus on landing a human on the moon by the end of the 1960s. The U.S. invasion of Vietnam led to radical movements and a rise in citizen power that sustained the decline in wealth of the richest 1% in the United States, to a low point in 1975.

We can rely on Kingdon's ideas framework to prescribe and dispense population medicine. We must end the apathy toward our health problem and present new ideas that will work to improve population health. This must be done *before* the next window of opportunity comes about, however, so that we're ready to push our policies into action and be well-prepared to make them function properly once implemented.

In considering that people in the United States have worse health than those in all the other rich nations some remedies might seem feasible. In yesterday's national climate, advocating redistributing income by means of higher taxation on the rich would have been political suicide. The U.S. 1.5 trillion dollar Tax Cuts and Jobs Act passed in 2017 reduced the top corporate tax rate from 35% to 21%. Not that many corporations paid the top tax rate, so the law was largely designed for an elite few. The Act, which in other decades would never have been seriously considered, was politically feasible because it was presented as paying for itself by spurring substantial economic growth, and would lead to higher wages, and decrease poverty. Did it produce any of those benefits? None.

Consider General Electric, one of our highly successful large corporations. In 2010, GE had worldwide profits of $14.2 billion including $5.1 billion on U.S. operations. Not only did they not pay any tax, but GE received a tax credit—a payment from the U.S. government—of $3.2 billion(13). This form of corporate welfare was all perfectly legal—and rewarded. The CEO of GE was named to head President Obama's Council on Jobs and Competitiveness.

President Biden wants to raise the top corporate tax rate to 28%, which is still considerably lower than what it was before 2017. But now may be the time to push for an even higher tax rate for these corporations. Given some popular politicians with socialist tendencies such as Senator Bernie Sanders and Congresswoman Alexandria Ocasio-Cortez, the Overton Window may have shifted toward taking higher taxation seriously.

Today there are many stories of big corporations, such as Amazon, paying no tax. Former President, Donald Trump, did not disclose his tax returns despite claiming to be a billionaire. He often did not pay any income tax. We may be entering a window of opportunity to raise taxes on the rich and wealthy corporations and maybe even consider a maximum wage although this is currently outside the Overton Window as politically unthinkable. On the other hand, raising the minimum wage is being seriously discussed.

Similarly, outside the Window is serious market regulation: a radical if not unthinkable possibility even though markets have caused so much misfortune. The so-called free market describes a buyer and a seller who negotiate a price to exchange goods and services. The seller includes his or her costs for producing the product and adds profit to the price. The buyer can offer a different price and in ideal circumstances they will come to an agreement and trade the product. The main issue here is that the seller's costs do not include what are called economic externalities. A simple example, I sell you a piece of lumber for your building project. The costs of this piece of wood do not include the destruction of the forest required to get it to market, nor the loss of carbon dioxide capture that this tree could have carried out. Nor the hazards of cutting the tree down, transporting it, and many other hidden costs such as habitat destruction that offers opportunity for animal infections to spread to humans. If all those were figured into the price you would likely find another solution to building a structure such as using an existing one, or not building a second or third home, or … Society, and in this case the planet, bears those external costs—and has led to our current global warming catastrophe and COVID.

Expanding public spending is now on the table. Proposals to boost the economy by rebuilding American infrastructure and forms of social spending are being considered in contrast to the Trump administration era. There is talk of a paid leave program, universal prekindergarten and free community college. Although raising taxes is being proposed as a way to pay for such programs, it will more likely come from using financialization, namely, borrowing money, and increasing the national debt which already is at its peak.

We must make the public aware of the problem. And major stakeholders have to agree on a feasible solution. Without the transforming event, not much will happen. Our task then is to create awareness of both the problem and possible 'medicines.' In Kingdon's process, ideas, such as our declining health status, really matter. But without awareness of the problem, little will change. The policy window can happen at any time, and when we recognize it, we must be ready to push our policy through. COVID could be this window today.

But we haven't yet done our homework to draw nationwide attention to the problem and potential solutions.

Conclusion

Producing a healthy population requires political action, first by creating awareness and considering novel 'medicines' and second, by being ready when a transforming event occurs. So just what are these economic and social remedies needed to restore American health? And what can we learn from other countries to help us answer that question? In the next chapter, we'll tackle those questions as we consider how to restore health in America.

Questions to Consider and Discuss

1. What opportunities exist today to shift the Overton Window and change the political contexts that shape our health?
2. Reflect on ways that your perception of reality has been altered by forces you were unaware of. How does advertising play into this? What can you do about these forces?
3. Consider the power nexus in your life. How much power do you have and how much do you want?

Notes

1. Yanis Varoufakis is a former Greek Minister of Finance and a founder of the Democracy in Europe Movement (DIEM).
2. John Dewey one of America's most prominent scholars in the first half of the 20th century—he argued that the attenuation of the shadow will not change the substance.
3. Attributed to Noam Chomsky, the most quoted living person today.

References

1. Rose GA. The Strategy of Preventive Medicine. New York, NY: Oxford University Press; 1992.
2. Steingraber S. Living Downstream: An Ecologist Looks at Cancer and the Environment. Reading, MA: Addison-Wesley Publishing; 1997.
3. Bezruchka S, Namekata T, Sistrom MG. Improving Economic Equality and Health: The Case of Postwar Japan. American Journal of Public Health. 2008;98(4):589–94.
4. Mendeloff J, Staetsky L. Occupational Fatality Risks in the United States and the United Kingdom. American Journal of Industrial Medicine. 2014;57(1):4–14.
5. Crozier M, Huntinngton SP, Watanuki J. The Crisis of Democracy: Report on the Governability of Democracies to the Trilateral Commission. New York, NY: New York University Press; 1975.
6. Carson-Parker J. The Options Ahead for the Debt Economy. Business Week. 1974; October 12:120–3.

7. Bernays E. Propaganda. New York, NY: Liveright; 1928.

8. Elgar FJ, Stefaniak A, Wohl MJA. The Trouble with Trust: Time-Series Analysis of Social Capital, Income Inequality, and COVID-19 Deaths in 84 Countries. Social Science & Medicine. 2020;263:113365.

9. Piff PK. Wealth and the Inflated Self: Class, Entitlement, and Narcissism. Personality and Social Psychology Bulletin. 2014;40(1):34–43.

10. Twenge JM. IGen: Why Today's Super-Connected Kids Are Growing up Less Rebellious, More Tolerant, Less Happy – and Completely Unprepared for Adulthood (and What This Means for the Rest of Us). New York, NY: Atria Books; 2017.

11. Kingdon JW. Agendas, Alternatives, and Public Policies. Updated 2nd ed. Boston: Longman; 2011.

12. Lynch J. Regimes of Inequality: The Political Economy of Health and Wealth. Cambridge: Cambridge University Press; 2020.

13. Kocieniewski D. G.E.'s Strategies Let It Avoid Taxes Altogether. New York Times. March 25, 2011.

Chapter 9

Prescription Needed

> We cannot solve our problems with the same thinking we used when we created them.
>
> *Albert Einstein*

If you live in the United States, your health has been compromised, particularly if you live in poverty, or if you are a person of color. Yet many may still be reluctant to accept this surprising feature of living in a nation that has been the global leader in wealth, technology and science, and human rights. Yet we are losing that lead, particularly in health and healthcare, something our response to COVID has made all too clear. What is wrong with our country, and what can we do to heal it? Before you can act, you have to critically evaluate what you have learned before reading this book, unlearn what is no longer valid, and then relearn.

Once you have discovered you are sick, then a diagnosis is needed; namely, you must determine what is the cause of your illness before you can consider what treatment is necessary. The same is true for a nation. This country is sick; namely, we do not have the health that would be expected for living in the richest and most powerful nation in world history. We die younger than people in more than 40 other countries.

The diagnosis is the extreme economic inequality we have together with the lack of support for early life. We have extreme wealth linked with immense poverty. The two are Siamese Twins. In most poor American communities, the disadvantaged do not complain of deep inequality. Instead, they focus on their own issues, namely, food and housing insecurity, inability to pay bills, lack of work, various illnesses they suffer from, and their lack of access to affordable medical care. They won't say, "Our problem is that the rich have too much." Their focus is downstream, related to tangible issues nearby.

The prescription needed is to shift our focus to the most upstream point of our model depicted in the illustration of Hawai'i.

In that model, we find socioeconomic status and above that political context and governance as upstream factors shaping our health. These factors are not ones our doctors will discuss with us. We have to formulate it ourselves from local ingredients.

DOI: 10.4324/9781003315889-10

Drawing attention to the compromised health status of Americans, together with strategies for overcoming the dysfunctional system that produces worse health are first steps toward this new understanding. The windows of opportunity for effective change are opening in today's nefarious political climate with its mis- and dis-information and fake facts. When the next transforming event occurs, we must be ready to push through policies to make America healthy again. Such a transformation is necessary not just in the United States, but in so many disadvantaged nations whose worse health threatens global survival.

What can we do to have better health?

Our CDC, the WHO, and other health organizations continue to focus on the individual, prescribing changes we can make in our diets, behaviors, and lifestyles. But as you have learned thus far in this book, these steps are not sufficient to facilitate the radical change we need for better health. Given what we have learned so far, what might the best tips be for good health?

They might be along the lines of:

- Be born in a caring, sharing, and repairing society.
- Nurture strong family and social ties.
- Don't be poor.
- Don't have poor parents.
- Don't work in a stressful, low-paid, and meaningless job.
- Don't live in a country with:
  - high income or wealth inequality
  - large health inequities
  - lack of time and resources for parenting
  - costly specialized inaccessible medical care.

Your doctor isn't the only one who will avoid discussing these issues. This counsel is not going to come from the public health professionals who advocate for more spending on medical care and public health to improve our well-being. Spending on medical care isn't that effective for producing good health. So let's consider social spending on policies that can promote better health and get us closer to following the tips above.

Social Spending

The Organization of Economic Cooperation and Development (OECD) was established in 1961 as a forum to stimulate economic progress and the market economy by making comparisons among member countries. The OECD now represents all the rich or developed nations along with several others. It is a statistical agency which compiles data on various categories from many countries. Taking a close look at some of the OECD data can give us a snapshot of how social spending relates to performance.

In 2011, health economist Elizabeth Bradley and her colleagues at Yale examined social expenditures and national health outcomes using OECD data(1). Social expenditures, both public and private, were characterized as old age pensions and support for older adults, survivors' benefits, disability and sickness cash benefits, family support, employment programs, unemployment benefits, housing support, and other social policy areas, excluding healthcare expenditures. Both healthcare and social expenditures were expressed as a percentage of the country's gross domestic product (GDP) in the relevant year.

The research team compared healthcare expenditures to social expenditures by country and found that most OECD countries spend twice as much on social expenditures as they did on healthcare. It was the other way around for the United States; we spent 25% more on healthcare than on social expenditures. The longer-lived countries with lower mortality target social spending rather than medical care spending. Countries with a higher proportion of social spending to healthcare spending enjoyed lower infant mortality and higher life expectancy.

Bradley's study has been replicated by others. One investigation considered California's social spending trends from 1990 to 2014. Of the total state budget in that period, social spending decreased by 13 percentage points, while healthcare increased by 7 percentage points. The study calculated that reallocation of spending from social to medical care in California resulted in 10,500 premature deaths over that period(2).

Government social spending is also much better at improving health than private spending. One study considered how much healthier the United States might have been in 2010 if it had the level of public social spending characteristic of other rich nations(3). In that study, considering OECD nations, the United States would have risen from 31st to 17th in life expectancy ranking. When poorer nations not in the OECD are examined, the United States standing drops even further to the level described in Chapter 1.

Another study looked at the social policy generosity in the OECD countries, considered as unemployment insurance, sickness benefits, and pensions. Beckfield and Bambra estimated that if the United States had just the average social policy generosity of the other 17 OECD countries, life expectancy would be over 3.7 years higher(4)!

The type of spending matters tremendously. Consider incarceration. The cost to the U.S. society is huge when we consider the expense of housing the highest number of prisoners in the world or to provide services for the homeless. One study looked at county spending on infrastructure (sewerage, fire protection, solid waste, and highways) as well as social spending (health, education, natural resource regulation, libraries, and parks) and showed health improvements, while there was no health benefit to spending on law and order(5).

The high rates of poverty in the nation constrain our society. We could take our own research, described in Chapter 5, and actively implement it, just as other nations are utilizing our results with successful outcomes.

The United States spends the least among rich countries on our children, their welfare, and inevitably their outcome as adults. The U.S. government spends $500 per child for care in contrast to some Scandinavian nations spending over 50 times as much(6)! The government of Sweden spends more on the first year of a child's life than in any subsequent year. Our expenditures focus on remedial efforts for social, behavioral, and academic improvement in the later childhood years. We are spending less proportionately than we did in 1960. As Frederick Douglass stated, we do not build strong children, but instead try to repair the broken men and women our neglected children become. We get what we pay for. We have failed our children. Is it too late to change course? Can we learn from Norway or Sweden's efforts to produce good health?

Why Might Sweden or Norway Be Healthier?

How did Sweden become considerably healthier than the United States? They are committed to social spending. Taxation rates are high, but the proceeds are returned to the people in the form of free education at all levels, early childhood education, free healthcare, very generous paid parental leave, and a variety of other benefits. Poverty rates are very low. The country provides resources to everyone so they can be free of dependency within the family and within civil society. When people are unencumbered by basic needs they can prosper.

Both Sweden and Norway have low income inequality. But wealth inequality—the unequal distribution of assets—in these countries is substantial, almost as much as in the United States. It has grown since the Great Recession in 2008. Reasons include a limited desire to save since almost all people have great economic security there. Norway does have a wealth tax. Despite these inequities in Norway and Sweden, the United States, with both its huge income and wealth gaps, stands alone among rich nations in its health-toxic economic inequality(7).

The key lesson to learn from Sweden is that the government provides the basics to everyone there so society can flourish. People recognize the benefits they all receive from paying high taxes. High taxation does not stifle creativity there (they file as many patents per capita as we do), an argument sometimes made in the United States to justify our extreme income and wealth differences. The Swedish government does not focus on changing individual behaviors to improve health, but on creating societal conditions so the population is healthy. They are less concerned with what individuals do or don't do to produce their health.

Compare taxation in America and Sweden. Over half of the Swedish GDP goes to the government, as taxes in comparison to only 30% accruing to the U.S. administration(8). In Sweden, the government expenditure goes to various forms of social spending. In the American situation spending goes to the military industrial complex, and to social security for older people. Our fiscal priorities do not produce good health.

Anu Partanen, a Finn, coined the phrase, "The Nordic Theory of Love." Nordic countries fulfill basic needs for their residents so they can be whoever they want to be. Such a philosophy enhances individual freedoms, rather than restricting them(9). This love is a common denominator in the Nordic nations. Similarly, in the paleolithic period everyone's basic needs were taken care of so they could be whom they wanted(10). But what accounts for the superior health in non-Nordic countries? Let's consider the nation with the longest life expectancy in the world. What did Japan do to become so healthy?

How Did Japan Become the Healthiest Nation?

You may be tempted to consider superior healthcare as the reason for Japan's exceptional health. Though everyone in Japan has access to healthcare through a universal insurance system, they have many healthcare idiosyncrasies. A few of these include considerably shorter doctor visits (due to their piecework doctor payment system) with doctors seeing on average over 75 patients a day. There are no required immunizations. Until 2005, there was no standardization of doctor and specialist training through competency examinations. Hands-on clinical training of doctors was very limited, yet these limitations have not shortened the lives of the Japanese.

Japan's good health status resulted after World War II. Japan was decimated after the United States fire-bombed Tokyo and later dropped atomic bombs over Nagasaki and Hiroshima. So many lives were lost that life expectancy plummeted to 24 years. The Allies then occupied Japan for 5 years. The head of the occupation, General Douglas MacArthur, wrote in his memoirs that Japan had been destroyed, and he wanted to rebuild its self-respect. He enacted three sets of policies, mostly enshrined in the Japanese Constitution that the Allies wrote for the nation. Article 9 abolished the military and required Japan to resolve all disputes peacefully. Other articles gave the country a democratic process, including women's suffrage, and free universal education. Another granted labor unions the right to organize and bargain collectively. Article 25 states, "All people shall have the right to maintain the minimum standards of wholesome and cultured living. In all spheres of life, the State shall use its endeavors for the promotion and extension of social welfare and security, and of public health." The United States promoted this progressive agenda of enshrining public health in the nation's Constitution—something we have yet to do here(11).

Before the War, Japan was run by 13 large family corporations, the *zaibatsu*. MacArthur recognized such concentrations of wealth and power structures would not promote democracy, so he broke them up. He legislated a maximum wage of 65,000 yen, and implemented an even lower maximum wage for the *zaibatsu* leaders. Similarly, 37,000 landlords (*jinushi*) owned the rice farming land (recall rice farming as a collective endeavor from Chapter 8) worked on by millions of tenants (*kosakumin*). MacArthur purchased the land at a fixed price per hectare, sold it to the tenants at the same price, and gave them a 30-year, very low-interest loan to pay for it. In the ensuing year, 94% of land changed hands in Japan. Historians call it the most successful land reform program ever. Japanese tend to abhor having loans, so most of them were repaid within a year. These redistributive efforts decreased economic inequality.

The resulting declines in mortality over this period were the most rapid ever seen on the planet. By 1978, Japan became the world's longest-lived nation. Japanese people welcomed these post-War changes presented in John Dower's Pulitzer prize-winning book, *Embracing Defeat*(12). The MacArthur "medicine" had three main ingredients: demilitarization, democratization, and decentralization (breaking up centers of power). This successful recipe could work in the United States, too.

The lesson Japan provides is that strong efforts to decrease economic inequality can produce rapid increases in health as measured by mortality. As we have seen with Russia and the Soviet Union in Chapter 3, rapid increases in inequality can produce the opposite—long-term declines in health. The United States needs to limit our recent rapid increase in income and wealth inequity so as not to prolong our health decline as happened in Russia.

What Is to Be Done?

You get what you measure. Or what gets measured gets done. Peter Drucker, the business management guru said, "If you can't measure it, you can't improve it." He also stated, "Management is doing things right; leadership is doing the right things." Given this definition, are we leading?

The most consistent indicators calculated every minute of every business day in this country are the stock market indices, the Dow Jones and the NASDAQ among others. They measure wealth creation. Increasing wealth is the focus in the United States. Wealth is by definition something only a few have. Just as we noted in Chapter 3, if everyone is poor then no one is, the same can be said of wealth—if everyone is wealthy, then no one is. Other prominent measures today are jobs and economic growth. The U.S. Department of Commerce reports the change in the GDP every quarter or three months. The U.S. Bureau of Labor Statistics reports employment figures every month. During the pandemic, COVID-19 cases are being tracked by various groups, including the CDC, and reported weekly. COVID internet dashboards report minute by minute. There is more information out there than we can comprehend, let alone track. We get what we measure most often, namely, wealth creation and COVID statistics leading to more deaths.

Let's define an index more relevant to those who are not attaining greater wealth. Rather than the Dow Jones Index, let's call it the Doug Jones Index to track how Doug Jones and his family are doing. Components of the index could include adult mortality in comparison to other nations, well-being similarly considered, status of their family housing, food security, adverse childhood experiences in their household, discrimination, and many other vital signs of a family in a population. All these data are presented in comparison to those in other nations. While the Dow Jones Index was telling us the economy is doing great, the Doug Jones Index tells us a very different story—Doug Jones' family isn't doing so well, not because he isn't working hard enough, but because they lack access to the resources necessary for an equal footing to enable his and his family's hard work to make a difference. We could track it in the major media daily, weekly, or at minimum monthly.

Except for a rare report in the media comparing our health status and whether it is improving or not, no federal body tracks our health in comparison to other nations. Once we track it we can improve it. The fact that we have more COVID-19 cases and deaths than any other country is also not common knowledge here. Once we and our managers (i.e., politicians) establish our health as important by measuring it, then we must get our leadership to improve it.

We must draw attention to our health not being what it could be because we live in the United States. This should be of concern to all of us, but to consider it requires challenging beliefs that have been strongly held since we were in our mother's womb. We steadfastly believe that personal behaviors and medical care produce health. How do such deeply held convictions change? In Chapter 1, we considered how someone comes to believe something is true. Notions become ingrained as common sense; namely, they do not need any evidence for us to accept them as true. Experience is also necessary to know something is true. Today social media can penetrate your sensory organs to experientially validate almost any belief without requiring any critical thinking skills.

Experiencing new concepts and understandings of what makes a population healthy is not easy. Circumstances in early life, the amount of caring we received then, are patterned by political decisions about how to share the society's resources. This means having a small gap between rich and poor that allows us to create conditions for a healthy early life. Social spending that benefits us from conception until we go to school is most important. Chapter 5 provides some conditions, such as paid family leave, and subsidized daycare, free preschool, and other societal supports that will impact the critical period for producing health in adulthood.

The Harvard philosopher John Rawls presented a theory of distributive justice implying fairness(13). He advocated everyone having the same basic liberties and a robust form of equal opportunity with the right of equal political participation. Inequalities in society should benefit the *least* advantaged. He described designing a society under a veil of ignorance meaning not knowing where you will end up. Thus, certain race/ethnicity, class, gender, natural endowments should not favor or disfavor outcomes. Under conditions of societal scarcity there must be enough to go around but not enough for everyone to get what they want.

How can we create such a society with its population health benefits that feature a small gap between rich and poor? To answer that question, let's explore income and wealth inequality in the United States beginning over a hundred years ago.

American Economic Inequality Trends

Recall the steep slope that led to so many people falling into the river that began Chapter 3. Is economic inequality the upstream or source effect mentioned in our earlier allegory? Is it the underlying problem that needs to be fixed? The answer depends on your political perspective. Many people today question the capitalist organization of society and the neoliberal transformation that has negatively impacted our lives in the last half century. Others believe there is no alternative to late-stage industrial state capitalism (meaning the state supports capitalism during its periodic crashes otherwise it would have self-destructed long ago) today. Progressives, however, speak vaguely of a post-capitalist world. It is more productive to rein in inequality in the short-term than to posit a nebulous concept of what the world might look like once we cast off the shackles of capitalism. How much inequality was there in the United States last century and how did it change during that period?

In 1913, the record gap in riches held by John D. Rockefeller and the rest of the 0.01% was 9% of American wealth. In 1929, the stock market crashed, and the Great Depression followed. The wealth gap dropped immensely to reach a low by 1975(14). Today the richest 0.01% of Americans hold 10% of all wealth, a record gap(15). We are far from Rawls' distributive justice. Our increasing mortality, whether from COVID-19 or other causes, is related to the vast U.S. economic polarization. In Chapter 8, we talked about how this divergence came about through adopting tenants of neoliberalism, namely, letting the rich have as much as possible.

What occurred in America after the Great Depression resulted from strong power of workers, through labor unions, and President Franklin Delano Roosevelt's (FDR's) efforts to save capitalism. FDR got New Deal legislation passed. These were a series of programs from 1933 to 1941 that provided social security, a minimum wage, a federal jobs program, banking safeguards, unemployment insurance, and other benefits. The power of workers is often overlooked as a part of this process. Union membership rose to 35% during this period. Powerful socialist and communist parties also pushed for greater equality. Democratic socialism operated in America then in contrast to fascist tendencies in Europe.

With the New Deal legislation presented by President Franklin Delano Roosevelt, a maximum wage of $25,000 was proposed in 1942 by having the highest marginal tax rate on incomes above that figure be 100%(16). When talking about this history of taxation I like to show people the April 28, 1942 *New York Times* front page with the lead headline, "$25,000 Income Limit ...

Asked by President." That amount then is equivalent to about $425,000 in purchasing power today. Most people could survive on that income. That legislation did not pass, but the bill approved by Congress in 1944 set the highest tax rate at 94%. In 1946, it was raised to 96%. In the 1950s, it was 91%. During the 1950s, incomes grew more for the lowest fifth of America than for the richest. The rising tide lifted the rowboats more than the yachts.

The top tax rate was lowered to 70% in the 1960s where it remained until the Reagan administration pushed it below 30%(8). That rate has had a few undulations to stand at 37% today—a far cry from 1946. The lowest tax rate has remained around 20% for this entire period. Meanwhile Western Europe has embraced democratic socialism as America has become increasingly protofascist. There were no protests against the high tax rates in the 1950s. They seemed fair to most people. While today a maximum wage is outside the Overton Window of Opportunity we discussed in the previous chapter, this could change.

How did we get from the small wealth gap between the 1940s and today's obscene situation? The richest have always wanted only one thing, MORE. They were not happy with their declining wealth share and their high tax rates. After World War II, the rich worked hard to change the political economy to get more. Organized labor power was decimated through legislation such as the Taft Hartley Act in 1947. In the 1950s, Senator Joe McCarthy exposed communists in the government, leading to the red scare that characterized any effort to protect workers as a communist plot. The Cold War that followed presented the Soviet Union as a convenient enemy out to destroy the American Way. The 1970s programs rolling out neoliberalism as an economic boom, actually punished the United States poor, who were stereotyped as the teenage welfare mother, or the ghetto street thug. As the poor were demonized and sent to prison (mostly for drug offenses), the wealthy were so admired they became effectively above the law, as the banking crisis of 2008–9 demonstrated when no one went to jail for those offenses. Instead, state socialism gave them bailouts and huge bonuses. By 2020, the unions once considered as a check on worker abuses, had become so demonized that union membership plummeted to less than 7% of private sector workers.

The rich made a concentrated effort to lower their taxes. A revolving door rotates between the Treasury and large accounting firms so Federal accountants can craft legislation to benefit the rich and get lucrative jobs afterwards. Many of the biggest American corporations pay no tax as they shelter their profits in off-shore tax havens and other legal means(17). Efforts to increase taxes, even on the rich, have been met with disdain by the general public. Until recently, the ordinary citizen supported tax cuts for the rich believing the savings of the rich would trickle downward. Whatever policies affected the rich, he believed, would ultimately affect him.

If we add up state and local taxes the situation becomes much more unfair. Back in the 1950s, there was not much of a spread in the top combined tax rate among the different income groups such as the bottom 10% of earners up to the top 90%. After that, for the top 10%, big tax rate gaps appeared. Consider the 400 highest income Americans and how much combined tax they pay as a percentage of their pre-tax income from 1950 to 2018. In 1950, the highest 400 individuals paid 70% of their income in taxes to the federal, state, and local governments. In subsequent decades the rate dropped continuously so that by 2018 they paid 23%, the *lowest* proportion of all income earners(18). By 2018, somebody in the bottom 10%, a worker with a pre-tax income of $18,500, paid 25.6% of that in taxes, in the form of local taxes such as sales tax, payroll tax, and property tax, so less went to the federal government. For the richest 400 Americans their taxes mostly went to the federal government. In Washington state where I live, as do two of the richest people in the world, Jeff Bezos and Bill Gates, there is no income or wealth tax but there is a high sales tax of nearly 10%. Since the ordinary citizen spends most of her or his income, they are disproportionately taxed; namely, they pay a higher rate of tax on much less income.

The public has mostly accepted their unfair burden, namely, paying proportionately more than the rich. This normalization of inequity was the result of the selling job described in the previous chapter. Such a tax system, where the poor pay so much more as a share of their income, is not only regressive but unjust. This extreme and worsening economic inequality is all pre-pandemic. It has likely worsened since the pandemic, given some of the pandemic profiteering discussed in Chapter 8 that has led to the current outrageous inequality.

Today's fractured societies can be seen as the political consequences of the grand deception perpetrated by the rich in the neoliberal tenet of letting the rich have as much wealth as they can. With today's extra-galactic inequality neoliberalism has clearly failed. People show their true feelings in practices such as the January 6, 2021, storming of the Capitol, and other forms of rage from political tribalism.

Today's challenge is to conceptualize economic inequality and its health impacts in plain language that will push people to rein it in. In Chapter 3, we portrayed the wealth of the richest person in stacked hundred dollar bills that reached over 120 miles into space. Such images help us consider different ideas. The mushroom cloud of an atomic or hydrogen bomb exploding commanded attention to considering a new form of energy. While we have seen the aftermaths of the destruction in Japan that two bombs caused, most of us cannot feel the real impact of that devastation. Nor do we see benefits from our landing on the moon. We become indifferent. The impacts of the global climate crisis make some of us feel uneasy, while feeling as abstract as the landing on the moon. But for many of us, global warming reflects personal stories such as evacuating when fires are burning, or moving to higher ground because of flooding, or being unable to farm because of drought.

The SARS-CoV-2 pandemic is similarly challenging for many to grasp. Like the climate crisis, it is an example of structural violence or social murder, something produced by missteps in leadership, individual misunderstanding, and unease with changing behaviors. It is probably no coincidence that both the climate crisis and the response to the pandemic in the United States are so fractured in ways that aren't present in many other countries. Just as other nations recognize the severity of the pandemic and acted pre-emptively when the United States did not, other nations recognize the severity of global warming and are taking action to stop it.

Why Do Americans Tolerate so Little Social Spending?

Recall how Scandinavian countries spend up to 60 times more than we do per person on childcare. Why? Why do we resist efforts to tax the rich even a little more than we do? Why do we not have more generous welfare supports as do the other rich nations? Why do we depend mostly on voluntary efforts to get the unhoused into shelters? And most fundamentally, why do we tolerate being dead first among so many nations?

We've presented some reasons such as our reverence for the wealthy. We seem inured to the plight of those lower down on the socioeconomic ladder. This has changed from having a focus on the middle-class portrayed on the 1970s TV sitcom show "All in the Family" or "Father Knows Best" from the 1950s to one of today's wealth portrayal of the obscenely rich. Examples are the serials "Succession" and "The White Lotus." Even the middle-class is portrayed as living in multi-million dollar homes. There are few movies or television shows that realistically portray the down-trodden who represent more than half of all Americans.

We are indifferent to the plights of many and distracted from their reality in our late-stage state-capitalism(19). What has led Americans to be so faithful to an economic system that has so failed almost all of us?

Harvard political economist Benjamin Friedman argues that religion plays a role in our understanding of modern Western economics. He gives three reasons for our unconscious belief in so-called free markets(20). The first he calls non-predestination thinking. We turned away from fatalism. Americans have been schooled to depend on their own ability and efforts partly as a result of Protestantism. The second comes from Protestant voluntarism. Our voluntary activities will take care of the needy. The third he feels comes from evangelical premillennialism; namely, when the rapture comes, the Second Coming, the future will result in blissful existence. And, they believe, it is just around the corner. All of us, not just the theists, are victims of these ideas.

The fundamental belief in American Exceptionalism prevents most of us from questioning whether we truly are the epitome of development(21). The question is, what are we going to do about it?

Steps to Reverse Our Intense Inequality

A window of opportunity to revise taxation is arising globally. Countries recognize that their tax base has been vastly eroded through various quasi-legal means that large multinational corporations use to evade paying taxes. The Pandora Papers revealing hidden wealth leaks released in October 2021 is another example. International meetings talk about establishing a minimum tax on corporations so they can't hide their profits and wealth. Such international tax reform discussions are not binding as we do not yet have a global financial system to regulate taxation. Nor do we have transparency. Many leaders talk about the need for such a system. In the aftermath of World War II, the Bretton Woods agreement led to creating an international monetary system. This lasted until 1971 when the United States ended the gold standard. If we consider that we are fighting World War III with the COVID-19 pandemic, we can push for an agreement so corporations can pay a fair share of taxes. Public support through political movements must foster such taxing power within each country. That means carrying out legislation in this country and cooperating with others.

Individual countries had difficulties providing social assistance to their people in the aftermath of the 2008–9 global banking crisis. They have cut services through austerity programs. As we see in the United States, however, this has not affected the richest 10% and especially the richest 0.01%. Various demonstrations and social movements in different countries have ordinary people calling attention to this plight. Consider the pre-pandemic Yellow Vest Movement in France. The Occupy Wall Street Protests spurred on by the 2011 Arab Spring uprisings and similar ones globally represent another. "We are the 99%" was their slogan as an awakening of democracy. The few in power fear people power so authorities evacuated the Occupy demonstrations. Effective protests come from people massing together physically and not from doing so on social media platforms, or emails or other virtual methods. Together, the power of we the people is much stronger than the power of the people in power.

A major difficulty in overcoming inequality, however, is that inequality has become normalized and ingrained in the U.S. psyche, at least since the 1970s. Unlike many political movements over the last few decades, there is no one culprit to focus on in contrast to other progressive efforts such as reducing carbon emissions, ending sweatshop labor exploitation, and enacting soda taxes. If one considers the arguments in Naomi Klein's *NO LOGO*, people prefer tackling more visible downstream issues(22). Similarly, other causes such as the United Farmworkers Union and the resulting lettuce boycott in the 1970s, the opposition to the invasions of Vietnam and Iraq, the War in Afghanistan, or the anti-fascist movements, have obvious villains to focus an attack. When individuals have strong views about their ideas, they come together, and the enemy can be revealed. Today, there is a huge wealth defense industry focused on advising billionaires on wealth hoarding(17). This trend is so extreme that in the next

20 years a minimum of $35 trillion (trillion with a T) and up to $70 trillion is expected to be inherited by the next generation—unless something is done.

A maximum wage would do more for our health than increasing the minimum wage, as whenever the minimum goes up, the highest earners get more substantial wage increases, and inequality increases. More equitable than raising the minimum wage would be a livable wage, enough to pay for food, housing, and other basic needs. Again, the mainstream media, owned by big corporations, are not doing much to push this process.

Consider a maximum wage as a form of economic democracy. While we may have political democracy, namely, the ability to choose our leaders, this does not exist in the workplace where the employers make the critical decisions. In some other rich nations, a substantial part of the board of directors of large corporations must be comprised of workers. In the 1950s and 1960s, CEOs made about 10–20 times what an average worker was paid. Today it is 300–500 times. One way to bring down top executive compensation is to incentivize corporations who pay their CEOs less as a portion of the median worker pay— the pay-ratio. Rhode Island, California, and Portland, Oregon have some form of this in process. Preferential treatment in bidding for government contracts for corporations with smaller CEO-worker pay ratios provides an incentive. Another would be a pay ratio surtax. This ratio can be monitored due to the Dodd-Frank legislation passed in 2010, which requires corporations to disclose their "pay ratio" (CEO compensation divided by that of the median worker) beginning in 2018. Pay ratio penalties for firms that pay CEOs more than 100 times what median workers receive are another option. Yet another would be graduated surtaxes on ratios of more than 250 times.

In Chapter 6, we saw how Blacks and Indigenous peoples do not have good health in America. Intergenerational transmission of historical trauma since slavery and colonization has limited health improvements of these groups. American progress today resulted from such exploitation so we have a responsibility for the sins of our forebears. Besides caring and sharing we must also repair. Reparations have taken place in many places around the world. William Darity Jr. proposes that we take excess White wealth in the United States today and transfer it so that African Americans who had one slave ancestor receive enough to eradicate the racial wealth gap(23).

Convenient Truths (or Side Effects) About Reducing Inequality

There are many benefits to decreasing economic inequality. These benefits include better mental health, less violence and, it turns out, decreasing the forces that produce global warming. In countries with smaller gaps between rich and poor, business leaders are more likely to comply with international environmental agreements. Such nations are more likely to recycle waste and produce lower CO_2 emissions(24, 25). American states, such as Delaware,

Maryland, and New Hampshire, that have limited the increase of the income share of the top 10% from 1997 to 2012, saw less CO_2 increase, and even declines in CO_2 emissions(26). Other studies demonstrate great social benefits in more equal nations. These benefits include less gambling and bullying, better math and literacy scores, higher adult educational outcomes, and higher trade union membership among the labor force(27).

Conclusion

We have within our reach many methods to potentially improve health in the United States. But these methods are broad public policies requiring social spending rather than offering individual advice. Policies and practices in healthier nations provide examples of what America could do. Attention must be drawn to Americans being dead first. Then we must set goals to end that carnage. U.S. economic inequality is at an all-time high but a window of opportunity to change that has arisen. Reducing this huge imbalance will profoundly benefit our health.

Stop for a moment and consider what you can do to improve health in this country. How can you contribute to raising awareness of the problem—and potential solutions?

How might you, the reader, take steps toward a healthier future now? How can you become involved in your community to improve your environment and social safety nets? What can you do to help change the laws and enact better ones to minimize income inequality and maximize social benefits? In the next chapter, we present some alternatives we must personally consider.

Questions to Consider and Discuss

1. The rich and powerful are threatened by the power of people. The 1930s New Deal came into being through popular organizing and produced policies that markedly decreased inequality. Does the Green New Deal offer similar hope for substantive changes?
2. What can be learned from healthier countries that might be applicable for the United States?
3. COVID-19 has disrupted everyone's lives. What will the new normal look like?

References

1. Bradley EH, Elkins BR, Herrin J, Elbel B. Health and Social Services Expenditures: Associations with Health Outcomes. BMJ Quality & Safety. 2011;20(10):826–31.
2. Tran LD, Zimmerman FJ, Fielding JE. Public Health and the Economy Could Be Served by Reallocating Medical Expenditures to Social Programs. SSM - Population Health. 2017;3:185–91.

3. Reynolds MM, Avendano M. Social Policy Expenditures and Life Expectancy in High-Income Countries. American Journal of Preventive Medicine. 2018;54(1):72–9.

4. Beckfield J, Bambra C. Shorter Lives in Stingier States: Social Policy Shortcomings Help Explain the US Mortality Disadvantage. Social Science & Medicine. 2016;171:30–8.

5. Cardona, C, Anand, NS, Alfonso, YN, Leider, JP, McCullough, JM, Resnick, B, Bishai D. County health outcomes linkage to county spending on social services, building infrastructure, and law and order. SSM - Population Health. 2021;16: 100930.

6. Mailler CC. How Other Nations Pay for Child Care. The U.S. Is an Outlier. New York, NY: New York Times; 2021 [cited 2021 6 October]. Available from: https://www.nytimes.com/2021/10/06/upshot/child-care-biden.html?smid=fb-nytimes&smtyp=cur&fbclid=IwAR0XDz8GxeI_lj3k8XLYzZA15cSM-sSQWfYRgXKzAi8OuanEaHiy8zBhg7g.

7. Lakey G. Viking Economics: How the Scandinavians Got It Right – and How We Can, Too. Brooklyn: Melville House; 2016.

8. Piketty T, Goldhammer A. Capital and Ideology. Cambridge, MA: The Belknap Press of Harvard University Press; 2020.

9. Partanen A. The Nordic Theory of Everything: In Search of a Better Life. New York, NY: Harper Collins; 2016.

10. Graeber D, Wengrow D. The Dawn of Everything: A New History of Humanity. First American edition. New York, NY: Farrar, Straus and Giroux; 2021.

11. Bezruchka S, Namekata T, Sistrom MG. Improving Economic Equality and Health: The Case of Postwar Japan. American Journal of Public Health. 2008;98(4):589–94.

12. Dower JW. Embracing Defeat: Japan in the Wake of World War II. New York, NY: W. W. Norton; 1999.

13. Rawls J. A Theory of Justice. Cambridge: Belknap Press of Harvard University Press; 1999.

14. Harvey D. A Brief History of Neoliberalism. New York, NY: Oxford University Press; 2005.

15. Wolff-Mann E. Super Rich's Wealth Concentration Surpasses Gilded Age Levels. 2021 [cited 2021 7 July]. Available from: https://finance.yahoo.com/news/super-richs-wealth-concentration-surpasses-gilded-age-levels-210802327.html?fr=sycsrp_catchall.

16. Kluckhohn FL. $25,000 Income Limit, Ceilings on Prices, Stable Wages, Taxes, Asked by President. New York Times. April 28, 1942.

17. Collins C. The Wealth Hoarders: How Billionaires Pay Millions to Hide Trillions. Cambridge, UK: Polity; 2021.

18. Saez E, Zucman G. The Triumph of Injustice: How the Rich Dodge Taxes and How to Make Them Pay. New York, NY: W. W. Norton; 2019.

19. Freudenberg N. At What Cost: Modern Capitalism and the Future of Health. New York, NY: Oxford University Press; 2021.

20. Friedman BM. Religion and the Rise of Capitalism. New York, NY: Alfred A. Knopf; 2021.

21. Lipset SM. American Exceptionalism: A Double-Edged Sword. 1st ed. New York, NY: W. W. Norton; 1996.

22. Klein N. No Space, No Choice, No Jobs, No Logo. New York, NY: Picador; 2002.

23. Darity WA Jr, Mullen AK. From Here to Equality: Reparations for Black Americans in the Twenty-First Century. Chapel Hill, NC: UNC Press Books; 2020.

24. Wilkinson R, Pickett K. A Convenient Truth: A Better Society for Us and the Planet. London: Fabian Society; 2014. Fabian Ideas 638.

25. Wilkinson R, Pickett K. The Impact of Income Inequalities on Sustainable Development in London: A Report for the London Sustainable Development Commission. London: Sustainable Development Commission; 2010.
26. Jorgenson A, Schor J, Huang X. Income Inequality and Carbon Emissions in the United States: A State-Level Analysis, 1997–2012. Ecological Economics. 2017;134:40–8.
27. Wilkinson R, Pickett KE. The Spirit Level: Why Equality Is Better for Everyone. London: Penguin; 2010.

Chapter 10

What Can We Do?

Knowing is not enough; we must apply. Willing is not enough; we must do.
Goethe

As I write this final chapter, COVID-19 has killed over a million Americans. It didn't have to be this way—hundreds of thousands of lives could have been saved. But political decisions prevented that from happening. Given our ineffectual response to COVID-19, how can Americans respond to future health threats? What can we do? What are you going to do with your one and only precious life?

The previous chapters described potential approaches for improving health in the United States, impacting various health determinants and focusing on the importance of inequality. Most books on making improvements stop at this point, as they have detailed the necessary elements that require changes. Here, we present many specific approaches to promote understanding and action both for stemming the health decline and fostering a healthy future for all. Nelson Mandela, the first President of Post-Apartheid South Africa pointed out: "Vision without action is just a dream, action without vision just passes the time, and vision with action can change the world." The British poet W.H. Auden, considering the destruction humans created in the Second World War put it: "we must love one another or die."

Key goals are to decrease inequality and support improvements in early life for every child born. We need three concurrent efforts: (1) Working as individuals and with others to better understand and address factors in the local environment that affect health; (2) Taking part in effective organized action to address the political structures that have made us one of the most unequal countries in the industrialized world; and (3) Raising broad public awareness of the fundamental role of inequality in determining our health, to develop a full-fledged social movement for change.

Alice Walker points out that the most common way people give up their power is by thinking they don't have any. We have power as citizens once we engage politically—and the time has come for a broad social movement that changes power relationships.

DOI: 10.4324/9781003315889-11

In this chapter, I present a variety of approaches on what you or your organization can do. We begin with a large range of actions to promote population health. We then ask, how might a broad social movement arise from these efforts? And what are the barriers to effective action?

Individual Efforts

The first step to making change is to find a relevant aspect of the inequality-health issue that resonates with you. The topics discussed here offer a wide range of issues for which effective action, taken together, will dramatically affect the health of this country. Perhaps it's the unfairness of our tax code, or the plight of those who struggle with two or three jobs at minimum wage and still can't afford housing, or the ways voting regulations constrain the participation of low-income or minority populations in your state.

You might decide to work on supporting a healthy early life for children born in America by promoting paid family or maternal leave. As a new parent yourself, you may have found juggling the demands of work and infant care stressful, both emotionally and financially. If your state already has a fledgling program—popularize it through social media. Work with grassroots groups and lawmakers to help other states enact such policies or campaign for a substantial national parental leave program.

Learn about whatever topic you choose in sufficient detail that you can provide useful, compelling information. With a grasp of basic information, consider what critics might say, such as a concern voiced by some on the right that "government interference" isn't needed. They frame the problem as one of personal choice: if women really want to stay home with their infants they can do so. Learn to voice reasoned responses to those concerns.

Find out what is happening locally. What organizations already support paid leave policies? Get involved with them and volunteer for whatever tasks may be needed. In Washington State where I live, the Economic Opportunity Institute drafted our State's paid family leave legislation and, once it became operational, it continues to work to make the benefits better known.

Inventory your skills and the activities you enjoy. If you are a musician, recognize that music has a way of speaking to many with powerful messages. Past social movements typically center around protest songs. Perhaps you are a meeting planner and like to organize events, or you enjoy networking and bringing others together. Maybe you enjoy organizing meetings on Zoom or using Slack to communicate within a group. You may be adept with social media skills and love Instagram. Use your doodling skills to create striking, informative graphics. Contribute your ideas and skills to the effort. They could include phone banking; contacting political officials to lobby for attention to early life; supporting a group's email list or web site; organizing public or virtual showings of important presentations on the topic, whether from speakers or videos, or a combination of both, or going door-to-door to support maternal leave initiatives. Creative groups develop a wide range of ways to promote their topic. Provide whatever financial contributions you're able to give as well.

Don't break the bank. Proceed on a low budget for efforts that you can personally afford. Often time is the key commodity rationed. Stemming our health decline will take a long time, even though we want fast relief.

I funded my own habit of drawing attention to the problems of population health by working in emergency departments. When I graduated from public health school in 1993, I was advised to not leave my "day job." It took me another 15 years to leave paid ER work. By that time, I was teaching university courses and supervising students, and earning enough. I enjoy teaching, writing, and talking. Organizing events—typically visits by renowned population health experts—is more challenging, but I arrange them periodically. I take to the street to demonstrate, although as I age that has become more difficult. Working with others who have different skills, collectively we can work synergistically for positive change.

Most of us carry technology with us that can capture quality video, audio, and photographs. Document important events taking place. Who knows how they might impact the world, the way the bystander video of George Floyd's murder did?

Here are some of the specific tools and approaches individuals can use to be actively involved in the quest for health equity.

Verbal Communication

Face-to-face communication has been the most common and effective information-transmitting technique. Communicate with people you see regularly or with a new audience, in individual conversations or something bigger, at a club or social gathering.

Your workplace is one effective way of having discussions on our health. While there has been a vast decline in labor union membership, in the past unions have been major forces pushing for progressive change, such as the New Deal. Labor unions are tailor-made for presenting the book's ideas though it is challenging to get their members to distinguish health from healthcare. Trusted co-workers and others may be eager to engage in conversations beyond "what did you do over the weekend?" I've done this with patients and families in the emergency department as well as the staff there. But be sensitive to know when to stop.

With many workplaces now virtual you can use this medium to some effect.

Many readers, particularly introverts, will not see themselves giving speeches or teaching courses. But it's possible to practice *acting* as an extrovert in order to better engage people. To gain public speaking skills and banish your fears, attend Toastmasters sessions. Toastmasters give you practice saying something meaningful, beyond what you did on your vacation. Introverted students who took that approach and were challenged by the experience went on to overcome their shyness and become compelling speakers. Effective oral presentations do require skills that can be developed(1).

Engage with people you don't know. Riding public transportation provides an opportunity to speak to a stranger and get comfortable with close proximity. Consider a small group doing real-life demonstrations at a bus stop that portrays country health. Walk instead of driving in your car. Approach people walking or sitting in public spaces, parks, or streets. Haphazard conversations with strangers can lead to substantive discussions. Discover what you have in common. Ask questions such as what they have been most curious about this week. Get to know the new parents you meet in your daily interactions. See if you can steer the conversation around to early life issues. When talking in a restaurant about these ideas, several times I've had someone at another table tell me that if I was running for office they would vote for me.

Consider street interviews with a video camera on a specific topic such as paid parental leave. Obtaining releases isn't necessary if done in a public place, otherwise get permission. We created such montages with that approach to demonstrate public support for paid leave that helped get legislation passed in Washington State.

Find your own ways of getting the listener's attention. When addressing a group formally, I often begin by asking, "What is the most serious sexually transmitted condition?" People volunteer a few ideas. I respond by telling them that "Everyone in this room is infected." The audience becomes uneasy. "Life is a serious sexually transmitted condition," I proceed. "You are all here because of a sexual act in which your father's sperm fertilized your mother's ovum that was made when she was inside her mother—your maternal grandmother." This gets a laugh. I then ask the serious question: "How are we going to treat this serious condition called life?" It's a great conversation starter. Use my ice-breaker in your group to start a dialogue.

I keep files of various phrases and speaking points I've used that jolt the audience, such as the one above. When I speak about early life, I begin with "As you go from the erection to the resurrection, the first thousand days matter most." Another is "early life lasts a lifetime." "We are dead first." "Inequality kills." Instead of calling them doctors, I say "MDeities." When you hear something that rings true to you, and gets an audience reaction, note it and put it in a computer file that can later be searched. Audiences are more likely to remember catchy comments than arcane statistics. And the media love sound bites.

I practice talks on our health status by recording them beforehand, listening to where the syntax isn't logical or words don't flow, and revising. When it comes time for the actual presentation, I don't read the speech but use an outline, recording each talk for later evaluation. With social media making us alone together, the future belongs to those who can talk face-to-face.

Telling a story is the best way to communicate. Personalize it. Make people feel an emotion. Try to expand your story to groups or even entire nations. Most stories are about individuals or at most a small group. You can make up your own story or find one in the media that illustrates an important point. In your talk make people laugh, make them cry and make them think.

Ask for feedback. Being open to comments, criticisms, and other perspectives is vital to getting better at explaining difficult concepts. Stand-up actors and comedians at improv performances quickly learn that some phrasings and jokes work but others don't. As a teenager I sold soft-drinks at a two-week long grandstand performance by Bob Hope, then perhaps the most sought-after entertainer. Every night his lines were exactly the same. They were all highly polished and very effective. Yet each night he sounded like he was presenting this material for the first time. Cultivate this skill.

There is a large industry out there engaging public speakers to give motivational talks to businesses and other organizations. Some of the people I have climbed with have used the mountain or adventure metaphor, strategies of getting to the top, to become successful inspirational speakers. Take on the challenge to craft such a presentation using the ideas in this book.

TED talks have potential for fostering awareness and understanding. A search for TED talks on income inequality and health reveals one by Richard Wilkinson on how inequality harms society that has received millions of views. More communities are organizing their own local TEDx talks. Apply to be one of their speakers. My two TEDx talks on inequality and health have had a respectable number of views. As you draw attention to our health status as a nation, people will often search your name out on the web. Having a TEDx talk under your belt gives you legitimacy. For inspiration search the TED space for inequality and health to hear what some say. Organize a TEDx event in your neighborhood.

Practice "elevator speeches"—short pitches, less than a minute—to spark conversation with someone as if you were riding in an elevator together. It's a requirement for my students. When the phone inevitably rings with a marketing call, they can turn the conversation from the caller's sales spiel to a rehearsal for the elevator pitch. The kind that starts with a disclaimer stating it's being recorded for quality assurance purposes works best, as the caller won't hang up. It's a great time to try your speech in your own words. Here's one example:

CALLER: Do you know your car warranty is about to expire?
RESPONSE: Do you know that for living in the U.S. we have worse health and
    die younger than people in over forty other countries? The length of our
    lives is declining and death rates are going up! Yet we spend more on
    medical care than any other nation in the world. What's wrong? One prob-
    lem is that we don't support early life, even though half of our health as
    adults is determined then. Only two countries don't have a national policy

to give working mothers who have a baby paid time off work. We are one, and the other is Papua New Guinea. I'm sure you're concerned, and I'd be happy to talk more with you.

TO FOCUS ON INEQUALITY, CONSIDER: Do you know that for living in the United States we have shorter lives and die before folks in over forty countries? Not because of our diet or medical care. Our income and wealth inequality are killing us as we die from the usual conditions such as heart disease, cancer, and COVID. The richest 400 people in America pay a lower rate of tax than you do. We can change that. I'd be eager to talk more about how.

It takes less than a minute to make such statements. Put it in your own words and practice in front of a mirror. Tell it to friends. Audio record the elevator speech and listen to the playback. Refine it. Asking "Do we want healthcare or actual health?" can start a discussion.

Meet with your elected local, state, or national representatives. Have a specific request for them to address. You can arrange a meeting by phone or on the web. Arrive with others that support your cause. Numbers count. Once, meeting with my congressional representative, I presented my ideas about the U.S. health through one of my elevator speeches. He listened intently and then asked how many others in his constituency felt like I do. Had I come with five others and had many more outside, the visible support would have made a bigger impact. Write letters to them, handwritten if possible, about the issues in this book. Physical letters make a difference, as most such communication today is by email. If you take the time to write a letter, rather than send an email, you often get a reply. Try to follow up on that, that is send another letter or ask to meet.

Podcasts have become popular. Consider starting a series on population health and recruit speakers. I've been recruited by people I didn't know to present material in this book. Showcase those who don't agree with your ideas. Consider a panel discussion among people who have contrasting points of view, challenging the listener to make up their own mind.

Recognize that many people in this country do not want to hear this book's message. Perhaps some of this resistance may be related to the widely-held belief that the United States is unquestionably the greatest country in the world. So many have internalized the American exceptionalism doctrine that they are unable to hear any facts that counteract that belief. They are indifferent. Or they may not like the way you present it. Be sincere and calm. Anger begets more anger, and a shouting match is bad for our health. Be as soft-spoken as you can. Present facts in reasoned prepared ways, using analogies wherever possible. I used to carry reprints of articles to hand out, but these days I send attachments by email.

As you gain confidence, find people who have different perspectives than those in this book. Engage in relaxed chatter and present a few ideas and listen to their response. They might express interest. Meet with them at different times over a substantial period. While you may not be successful in changing their perspective, sometimes you might.

Graphics

Visuals or graphics are absent from the best speeches except for the biblical one using two stone tablets. But today effective graphics help convey some messages. Facebook or Twitter postings without a compelling graphic are more likely to be ignored. Attention-grabbing visual portrayals of our nation's health status related to other countries are needed. We need to develop videos that go viral demonstrating issues such as the deterioration of our health over the years. An image of someone slumped over from an opioid overdose might garner attention, but it would then focus on needing to treat the addiction rather than explaining why we consume more opioids than any other nation. On the other hand, having a photo of a "Pain Institute" near where two of the richest people in the world reside and asking why we have so much social pain makes a novel connection.

A map of the United States and Canada depicting life expectancy in different colors among states and provinces is informative but unlikely to catalyze change. The impacts of rising inequality are delayed, and they are distant, over there, not here. Perhaps focusing on deaths of despair is more meaningful. A picture of a dead and decaying albatross with plastic materials where its stomach used to be, or a beached sperm whale that ate 64 pounds of plastic, may affect people so much that they may consider reducing their use of plastics. Bystander videos of policemen shooting retreating, unarmed, young Black men have created a movement advocating for more responsible policing. After the police murder of George Floyd in the summer of 2020, the Black Lives Matter crusade went global and remains a compelling force today. You've seen many similar examples. Produce creative graphics as a visual depiction of our health decline.

Income inequality is easier to portray than declining health. Professor Ichiro Kawachi at Harvard, mentioned in Chapter 3, uses depictions of freshly minted hundred-dollar bills arranged into stacks to represent the incomes of the richest members of society. When he speaks about how income inequality affects health, he portrays a stack of hundred-dollar bills that represented one person's annual income of four billion dollars. In Seattle, he showed a picture comparing this stack of bills to the summit of nearby Mt. Rainier (14,411 feet), to demonstrate how high those bills would reach (4 billion tops out near the summit). Near Washington D.C., Kawachi uses the Washington Monument to reference how many of monuments must be stacked to represent the same amount of money. His locally relevant and memorable visual depictions say far more than words.

Pictures help communicate. I photograph billboards with important messages. One in Bothell, Washington, said, "You think smoking kills? Try working a dead-end job." It was an attention-grabber, pitching a job-finding website.

One from the early 1980s set in Oakland, California had the text, "Stress at work? Powerlessness is bad for your health." The response was to call a phone number for stress and family counseling. When I present this billboard photograph, I point out the individual response to a societal issue. Such images are opportunities to get discussion going.

Take photographs depicting inequality in the world around you. Doing so will help you sense our various overt and covert power structures. Show the wealth divide by photographing public schools in poor neighborhoods with private schools in wealthier ones. Take a wide-angle view of a homeless shelter with the financial district towering in the background. A street vendor outside a designer store. Demonstrators fighting inequity. Share these images on social media.

One student created a graphic using the common biohazard symbol with flaming red text overlay stating, "Economic Inequality is Hazardous to Our Health." She sells T-shirts, buttons, mugs, postcards, and stickers with this graphic on her website. I keep this image on the backside of my clipboard, so when I am talking to people, I can hold it in front of me with the biohazard symbol facing them, subtly drawing attention to the concept. A student group produced a button picturing a prescription vial that had the lettering, "Reduce the gap between the rich & the poor. Warning: may cause good health." Gather your own arsenal of powerful images, and post them on social media. Engage in the discussion that follows.

Whatever you do, recall what P.T. Barnum said: "without promotion, something terrible happens ...... nothing."

Institutional Outreach Efforts

In medical school I produced an "Absurd Drug Ad of the Month" poster, and placed it in a main hallway. Each month I would place a drug ad from a medical journal there and use it to inform about the drug industry. Think about what type of poster you might display where you work—though you may need to get permission from administration.

For those with the power to set examination questions or develop curricula for schools, many possibilities exist to enhance our understanding of U.S. health. Consider standardized testing such as the various state exams during grade school, SAT (Scholastic Aptitude Test) for college admission, GRE (Graduate Record Examination) for graduate school admittance, MCAT (Medical College Admissions Test) for medical school entry, LSAT (Law School Admission Test), etc. There are medical licensing exams, both for getting a credential to practice in a state as well as attaining specialty qualifications. If those tests had questions about U.S. health status in comparison to other nations, then this material would be taught, either through the review course industry, or in educational curricula.

What kind of questions might encourage people to reflect on the issues raised in this book?

Those teaching in medical schools, nursing schools, or the social sciences have opportunities to cover material about health inequities, health systems, and population health. While inroads have been made to incorporate population health concepts, these and public health topics tend to be slighted in the already overcrowded curriculum. To make these ideas more acceptable call them social medicine(2). The critical issue with all of these terms is to actually discuss health in the United States in comparison to that in other nations.

Executives or administrators in an organization who have followed the concepts in this book thus far, will have their own ideas on how to raise awareness of U.S. health status in that institution. Internal newsletters come to mind, as do lunch meetings, and web rambles such as that mentioned below. Presently, Diversity, Equity, Inclusion (DEI) trainings and workshops are common in organizations. We need to come up with a similar strategy concerning U.S. health.

Public Demonstrations

Many events gather stakeholders on various issues and march through the streets or protest in front of buildings or gather in public spaces. Attend those that interest you and draw attention to population health. I wear a blue baseball cap lettered: Make America Equal Again. For one of the World Trade Organization (WTO) protest days in Seattle I marched with a hand-lettered sign on a stick saying, "WTO Makes Us Sick." A media person saw the banner and asked me to come speak to a radio station table covering that event. At other demonstrations a group of School of Public Health faculty held a cloth banner in front of us with a population health statement. Demonstrations by the Washington Physicians for Social Responsibility (WPSR) typically have the marchers wear white lab coats—the costume doctors wear. Large gatherings in public demonstrations are the bedrock of democracy. Governments fear them. But consider the successful efforts in Sri Lanka where people occupied the presidential palace to force the government out. That didn't solve the problem but directed global attention to people power.

Video Presentations

If public speaking is not your forte, be active in public venues by screening and discussing one of several compelling documentaries. Two good examples are the films *Unnatural Causes: Is Inequality Making Us Sick?* and *The Raising of America*. These videos are available from public libraries or from the *California Newsreel* website. That website contains suggestions for successfully organizing an event, doing a screening, and discussing the material. Before COVID-19 my students were required to do a community outreach activity in a place to which people were invited. They presented segments of one of the videos and fostered a discussion. Besides showing these excerpts, they could engage in other creative ways. Some realized that the material was both interesting and new to many of their audience members so would continue doing presentations afterwards.

Another catalyst for raising awareness is Michael Moore's documentary *Where to Invade Next*. Moore visits various countries in Europe and North Africa to show a range of social policies that could be implemented here. Some of the topics explored are humane conditions in Norway's prisons, Iceland's response to their banking crisis, sex education in Finland, and how French grade schools provide five course school lunches. Many eye-openers for meaningful discussions.

Social Media Efforts

The reach through social media is an excellent opportunity to build a platform for your message. Consider an Instagram or Google Forms survey, posts on Facebook, TikTok videos, and more. There are many ways of using your creativity here. Create a Facebook group on population health. You'll find plenty of information on how to do this on their website.

Playing Games

Consider playing the board game *The Last Straw: The Social Determinants of Health* that engages people in discussing these concepts. Mimicking life's experiences, the game begins with developing a profile at birth, rolling dice to determine each player's gender, socioeconomic status, and race profile. Players proceed around the board, traveling through childhood, adolescence, adulthood, and old age. The game requires discussing determinants and ways to adapt to various community issues from early life onwards. Those who start with a lower socioeconomic status (receiving fewer "vitality chips") don't do well. The game works for anyone over age ten. Players find it entertaining and informative. Medical schools in Canada use it for teaching. A web search for "The Last Straw Board Game" will locate it. It can be adapted to the online space.

An environmental game used in my classes is long remembered by students. The class is arranged into four or five groups, identified as regional communities or nations, who sit together to discuss which group will be chosen for receiving a load of toxic waste. Each group is given information about their health and wealth status as well as demographic details. Typically, others vote to give the waste to recent immigrants or a poor powerless country. These are the voiceless groups whose language barriers required they not speak when called upon, so they couldn't make the case for it going somewhere else. This memorable game, invented by Linn Gould who founded Just Health Action, helps students understand power relationships.

Play the world's best-selling game, Monopoly, with different rules to illustrate the inequities of our economic system. For example, one player follows normal rules, the second goes to jail for rolling a number higher than seven, the third only moves half the amount on the rolled dice, and the fourth twice the roll, etc. Creative versions of the game are available. On the internet search for *The New 'Monopoly' Rules for an Unfair World*. *Cheaters' Monopoly* and *Monopoly Socialism: Winning is for Capitalists*. Online versions are available including those that can be played on a smartphone. Another is the Money Game, played in rounds with different rules about giving or receiving real money. Look for rules on the Population Health Forum's website under the "Resources" link. None of the Monopoly games make links to health issues as does *The Last Straw*. Invent your own game to get people to grasp serious health issues.

Venues

Where can you present your ideas? Your church, your club or organization, the workplace, a gathering of friends, the local library, or political events you attend are possibilities. Consider local colleges; teachers are often looking for interesting presenters. When Richard Wilkinson spoke at a Seattle Town Hall event we scheduled several follow-up discussions in local libraries and prepared a bookmark with the dates and places that was placed on each seat beforehand.

Teachers at almost any educational level can present these ideas to students. As you gain skills doing this, consider producing a MOOC (Massively Open Online Course), through Coursera, edX, or some other platform. Ichiro Kawachi's MOOC has garnered more contacts for him throughout the world than any other effort.

Seek out creative retirement centers and give talks or put on courses for older folk. These venues are ideal audiences, as they have a lifetime of experience to draw upon that younger people lack.

Doctors and other healthcare workers can discuss this book's social medicine ideas with patients and their families. I did this with selected patients in the emergency department. Primary care doctors have an advantage, as they can discuss poverty issues and strategies for protecting incomes. One Toronto family doctor who treats poverty as a disease has inspired others in Canada by developing a clinical tool for addressing poverty. Besides taking a specific social history, he has various resources that patients can use. A family doctor working with marginalized patients near Seattle has developed a brief intake survey on social determinants containing just a few simple questions. What is your stress level? Are you homeless? Did you eat yesterday? Are you working/ studying? Can you read and write in any language? Can you speak English? Such a social history establishes a baseline from which to work.

Andra, a former student, produced and piloted a population health curriculum for a grade six class. Students learned about the importance of social factors, such as the idea that eating fast food was not the basic reason children became fat, but that it was rather the result of more upstream forces. One student said, "Before, I thought there was something wrong with those people. Like, why would you want to become a teenage mom when you don't even have an education? But now I see they don't really have a choice." Don't underestimate what young people can understand.

Middle and high schools are important venues for population health education. I've honed my skills in engaging the students' critical thinking skills without committing PowerPoint malpractice, showing no visuals at all. One creative homework exercise is to have students graph the top 20 country life expectancies. Curious students will continue the graph until the United States shows up! As we saw in Chapter 1 early exposure to ideas by those you respect, reinforcement by peers and authority figures, are key elements of acquiring knowledge. We need to assure that young people are exposed to these ideas when their attitudes and beliefs are forming(3).

Do a Population Health Web Ramble. I use a standardized series of instructions that get students to peruse websites and discover how we are doing in mortality comparisons with other nations. I begin with a quiz developed for the documentary series, *Unnatural Causes: Is Inequality Making Us Sick?* mentioned above, which aired in 2008. Ten internet questions have answers appearing right away, although the data are old, and our health has deteriorated considerably since then. People are surprised by what they learn. Next, they go to the Institute for Health Metrics and Evaluation website to look county life expectancy data for the United States as in Figure 6.2. Next, they look at the child and adult mortality site where they can put in nations around the world and see trends. I give them countries such as Sri Lanka, Peru, Tunisia, and others to compare with the United States. As in Chapter 1, they can calculate how many fewer children would die every day in this country if we had Slovenia's child mortality rate. They write up their findings as well as their personal responses to the discoveries. When this exercise is part of a course and they get a grade, it gets done. Without that requirement only very interested people will complete it. Contact me if you want an example via StephenBezruchka.com.

Another way with a group in a virtual breakout room, or sitting around a table, has them sort a dozen cards with country names on them for a health indicator such as life expectancy, or maternal mortality from the highest (best) to lowest (worse). They don't use the internet or outside resources. After recording the sorting, they do it again, this time with the internet to discover the correct values and order. They present this information to others. Your job is to choose the country names, and indicators to make valid points. Ideas abound(4).

College students can join student public interest research groups (Student PIRGS). Search them out and work together.

Media

Talking about notables who live to a very old age is another way of pointing out what we don't achieve. Highlight that the "oldest old" person at any one time on the planet is almost never an American (they typically hail from Japan). Ask an audience which prominent Americans they know who died before reaching age 60. Listeners may recall these ideas later and reflect on the grim prospect of dying young in America.

Community resources, including local low-powered radio stations, often look for inspiring content. Search for these local stations and contribute to content exploring local topics using critical thinking. If you're media-savvy you could also publish an online community newsletter or blog, or simply respond to blog posts. A group of Seattle colleagues produced a spoof of a local paper, entitled *New Clear News*, with fantasies about our undertaking nuclear disarmament. Every community needs inspiration to imagine what could be. Other resources to help you include the Berkeley Media Studies Group, The Pulitzer Center, and The Story Center.

The Written Word

Countless outlets for the written word range from letters to the editors of newspapers, to blogs, listservs, and social media posts. Explore possibilities with publications you have access to through your work, your hobbies, or organizations you belong to. Many are looking for fresh material from readers. Write letters to your congressional representatives and other officials who have the power to support the changes you are seeking. In this digital age, original, handwritten letters are still one of the most effective ways to let him or her know your opinion, second only to showing up in their offices for a discussion.

Op-Eds, substantive essays posted opposite the editorial page of newspapers, can call attention to population health issues. Those most likely to be printed will take advantage of local events to draw the reader in. Steps include: (1) Craft a succinct title that draws immediate attention to the key idea, since your title is your first, and often only, chance to catch viewers' eyes; (2) Hone your message into a few main points and limit data to one or two essential facts; and (3) Attention spans are short these days, so aim for a 750 word limit. Relate your op-ed to a current news story and personalize it.

Organizational Efforts

Consider major changes both in the United States and around the world that might have once been considered impossible, but happened because of strong efforts by organizations—such as the example of getting rid of lead in paint and gasoline. There are similarities to our current hazardous inequality situation. At the turn of the 20th century, a paint manufacturer pointed out the dangers of leaded paint. Nothing happened then, but after so much evidence appeared on its harms and those of lead in gasoline, the U.S. government banned lead-based paint in 1971. Blood lead levels can be measured and are still found to be high, especially in poorer folk. Overall the situation is improving. Lead abatement programs continue today. Leaded gasoline was last sold in Algeria until 2021. This required the participation of governments, non-governmental organizations and others operating under the United Nations Environment Program. Our world is still coated in lead but progress is being made to remove the metal.

Consider the similarities with reacting to our killer, economic inequality. We can monitor health outcomes among populations and pass legislation to decrease inequality. Progress can then be monitored to demonstrate decreasing gaps in life expectancy around the globe.

The African proverb, "If you want to go fast, go alone. If you want to go far, go together," bespeaks the need to form coalitions and mobilize communities for effective action. Individual efforts need to be combined with the efforts of committed groups that coalesce around common themes and actions. These backbones of collective activity can be both virtual and face-to-face but the most effective are face-to-face. Here are some ideas about how we can "go together," from the international level to the regional and local.

International

Consider the People's Health Movement, Occupy, Black Lives Matter, Socialist Forum, #MeToo, 350.org, Extinction Rebellion, and Democracy In Europe Movement 2025 (DIEM25), as examples of templates for developing one to decrease the mortality differences between nations. The highest are those in Sub-Saharan Africa and the lowest in Japan and Western Europe. The World Health Organization should have such a goal.

National

Surprisingly few efforts are apparent today at the national level that focus on upstream strategies to stem our health decline. The American Public Health Association (APHA) should be an ideal candidate, although to date it has mostly led with slogans, such as our becoming the "healthiest nation in one generation." Many of its subgroups such as "The Spirit of 1848" do remarkable work. A group of us got a resolution linking income inequality and health passed at the annual meeting of the APHA. The effect may be minor but working with others to accomplish this can build coalitions. Consider such efforts in organizations you belong to. Occupational associations such as those for doctors, nurses, pharmacists, teachers, and many others present good opportunities

The federal CDC previously had any relevant efforts curtailed by the Trump administration, and today has little power. Massive defunding and declining staff morale there limit CDC discussions of the U.S. health compared to other nations. A growing number of healthcare organizations recognize and aim to address social determinants of health, but efforts mainly champion individual determinants without expressly urging political action. Mainstream academia is mostly focused on research on specific medical issues or healthcare approaches and always drawing attention to the need for more studies. But we know enough to act.

A major impediment to organizations working to stop our health decline is their equating health with healthcare. Our health decline began with the implementation of the Affordable Care Act, which gave more people access to healthcare. The simple fact that treating our medical problems, even doing it well and for everyone, will not by itself makes us healthier is a reality to confront. Yes, access to healthcare is an important basic human right, and we should fight for it. No, it will not stem our health decline, and we must aim for the larger goal of increasing equity to make us have the health we deserve.

National level efforts ultimately have the greatest promise of changing our current downward trajectory in health. Their support is important for our work. A basic principle is to strengthen the public sector to counter corporate influences such as public-private partnerships whose goals rarely decrease inequality or substantially support early life. Government has been characterized as the problem, rather than the solution. That aphorism must reverse. Strong democracies make it easier to change distributions of wealth and power. Ending Americans being dead first requires protecting democracies.

Richard Wilkinson and Kate Pickett, key researchers in our story, started *The Equality Trust*, an organization in the United Kingdom when they launched *The Spirit Level*. It focuses mostly on the issues there but has much useful global material on its website.

More equitable taxation is a key important approach to reducing our rising inequality. A few well-focused groups that have newsletters providing updates and opportunities for action include: *Tax Justice Network* is an international group founded in the United Kingdom that focuses on educating about global tax injustice; *Tax Justice Now* considers the United States; *Inequality.org* provides analysis and commentary on income and wealth inequality, and produces an insightful weekly newsletter; The *Institute for Policy Studies* is a think tank that educates on a number of progressive issues. For workplace democracy concepts I subscribe to Richard Wolff's Democracy@Work series through Patreon. These videos are available directly on YouTube without having to pay but such work should be supported financially.

Find a national group that supports your specific social or health interest. Public health workers could work with the activist organization *Public Health Awakened*. The *Coalition on Human Needs* is a national alliance that has a huge list of groups focusing on poverty-related issues that work together. Four principles of their legislative work are to: (1) protect low-income and vulnerable people, (2) promote job creation and strengthening the economy, (3) increase revenue from fair sources, and (4) seek responsible savings from wasteful spending in the Pentagon and elsewhere. Progress in any one of these areas would support a more equitable country, which would in turn contribute to improved health.

Consider joining the national or local efforts of the *Poor People's Campaign*. Set up by Dr. Martin Luther King Jr. in the 1960s, the campaign's aim was to mass hundreds of thousands in D.C. and lobby elected officials for an economic bill of rights. Today they rise under a National Call for Moral Revival and focus on 140 million poor and low-income Americans. Get involved in one of the branches in many states.

You will find a national organization to help you learn and take action. For example, *Zero to Three* has a plethora of resources for those who wish to focus on support for a healthy early life. Another is *ThousandDays* with an international outreach. *The Living Wage Network* helps communities increase and strengthen recognition of employers who pay a living wage to all employees. Join, get involved, and contribute as you can.

Regional and Local

Organizations close to home provide the benefits of more person-to-person activism. I joined the Washington Physicians for Social Responsibility's Board of Directors in 2014 to help create an economic inequity health task force. (Don't be put off by the name of the organization, as most members are not physicians.) WPSR carries out a range of activities that were traditionally focused on nuclear weapons concerns, but now also include global warming and the inequality-health relationship. Our task force has carried out training sessions on promoting greater public and political awareness of the U.S. health status, and we were also part of a successful effort to pass state legislation providing for paid parental leave. Find organizations in your area supporting paid family or parental leave, such as the Economic Opportunity Institute in Washington State. Look for state partners at the *Center on Budget and Policy Priorities* for the relevant agency.

Find organizations near where you live or work to work on inequality and health. These could be church groups, temples, synagogues, or mosques, or perhaps carpools, community gardens, or reading groups. Post an organizational start-up meeting announcement in your local library or community center and publicize it widely. Schedule a regular "meaningful movies" night in your community on relevant topics. Draw attention to our declining health by whatever means available such as hand-lettered yard signs, bumper stickers, or buttons, but remember to link it with health, not healthcare. My favorite bumper stick says "don't believe everything you think." People have approached me after reading it.

For effective local action, investigate the aims of any promising-sounding groups you hear about. Once you become familiar with one such group, others working toward common interests will emerge. Decide which one best fits with your interests and skills and join up.

A Social Movement

You're only one person, so you can't do that much. But so is everyone else. Don't be one person! People working on critical, timely issues as individuals and then together with those others is how social movements begin. These phenomena have influenced how our culture evolved. Movements all start small, as renowned anthropologist Margaret Mead said, "Never doubt that a small group of thoughtful, committed citizens can change the world. Indeed, it's the only thing that ever has."

Large-scale efforts to address our increasing mortality are beginning. We've not yet had deniers of our health decline. The dead (mortality statistics) don't lie. At this point, increasing mortality is mostly an American phenomenon; before COVID-19 we were about the only industrialized country seeing increased death rates. There is no "Make America Healthy Again" action cry yet.

Recall the Hawai'i Dept. of Health mountainside graphic; the first approaches that come to mind for improving health are aimed at downstream effects: promoting healthcare and getting individuals to modify personal behaviors. That is where the river's current has taken us. But such work has been carried out for decades, and our current state of health status decline shows these efforts have by themselves been grossly inadequate. At the waterfall are the social determinants, focusing on improving conditions that produce health. Finally, at the upstream source of root causes, are the political issues that affect those social determinants. An active, relevant, and effective social movement for health must include this level, while not minimizing the more downstream factors.

The climate crisis response presents approaches that may be effective in fostering a social movement for health equity. Efforts to create awareness of global warming have been ongoing for more than twenty years. Vice President Al Gore drew attention to the crisis with his 2006 Oscar-winning documentary, *An Inconvenient Truth*, depicting his lecture circuit efforts to raise awareness on climate disruption. Many of the early ideas on how to respond, however, focused downstream, such as urging individuals to use more efficient lightbulbs. In the intervening years, greater awareness and activism around the world have moved the focus far upstream. For example, many countries signed onto the Paris Agreement in 2016 to voluntarily mitigate global warming by reducing its primary causes. Most nations have made efforts, with some progress. COP26 is the latest step. Young people, such as Greta Thunberg, will be the most impacted by global warming. They have mobilized in major ways. Read books on organizing movements(5–9). The climate justice movement, albeit with a slow start, is now well under way as a result of youth activism. Learn their techniques and transfer them to population health issues(10).

Past social movements have used a variety of techniques ranging from protests and blockades to the mass mobilization seen in the abolition and civil rights movements. In the 1700s, women in New England, concerned about slavery, wanted to draw attention to its brutality. They formed "sister societies," speaking at community gatherings about the ills of slavery(11). Their efforts spawned the abolition movement that long afterwards ended slavery.

The social movement for suffrage grew out of the abolition movement. Suffrage for women was limited to White women. A former slave, Sojourner Truth, spoke out publicly in 1851 saying, "Ain't I a woman?" Some of the key leaders had also fought against slavery, such as Susan B. Anthony and Alice Paul, both Quakers. To draw attention to their cause, the suffragettes launched fashion trends. Some ran for political office—despite not being allowed to vote. They also joined forces with similar movements in other countries. Success came in 1920 when women gained the right to vote in the United States. Blacks were guaranteed the right to vote after 1965. Some 15 states had already granted women voting rights before it became federal law. States can lead the way.

Social movements are becoming more visible each year. A 2015 U.S. Supreme Court decision legalized same-sex marriage following grassroots action for gay rights. Other efforts have provided a range of protections for the LGBT movement that were unthinkable just a few decades ago. The history of progressive social change is inspiring, and not the work of individuals. Progressive change requires a social movement for success. Audio cassettes catalyzed the Central America political uprisings that produced massive physical protest.

The Arab Spring in 2011 prompted a series of protests, movements, and rebellion against oppressive governments in the Middle East organized on social media that led to massive numbers protesting in public, especially at Tahrir Square. It birthed an effervescence of rebellion which was suppressed by the powerful few. The movement will rise again.

A single event involving one person can catalyze a global movement, just as Rosa Parks' refusal to give up her seat on a bus propelled the Civil Rights Movement forward, the killing of Matthew Shepherd fueled gay rights movements, Erin Brockovich spearheaded legislation protecting consumers from exposure to industrial toxic waste, and George Floyd's murder launched the Black Lives Matter movement.

Charity or solidarity? The rich and powerful create philanthropies to throw crumbs at us, and they decide which scraps to toss. Philanthropy exerts power over public life. Meanwhile the wealthy enrich themselves rapaciously, as we have seen with COVID. Activism and solidarity must become a normal activity throughout society, rather than something only a few engage in. Numbers matter. If one percent of the American public focused on our staying alive longer, that would compel the powerful to acquiesce, especially once they recognized they would live longer. This would lead to interdependence rather than hyper individualism, reciprocity rather than dominance, and cooperation rather than hierarchy. This challenging goal will be politically realistic after a few more catastrophes. Grow rice instead of corn to reflect the shift in cultural values!

Major economic shifts are essential to address our health decline. Those changes will require a broader awareness of the effects of upstream factors on our health. The groundwork is being laid: public resistance to our increasing inequality is growing, with disaffected Americans recognizing they are being exploited by the sick system. Our future work needs to focus on exposing the ways in which rampant social injustice affects not just our economic well-being but our prospects for a healthy life. Inequality kills!

Overcoming Indifference

We have looked at large numbers of people constrained by geography or socio-economic status and considered as our health measure mortality rates. Mother Theresa, who received the Nobel Peace Prize for her work assisting those dying in Kolkata, India said: "If I look at the mass I will never act. If I look at the one I will." We respond to individual stories of tragedy and need. Consider the success of Go Fund *Me* campaigns. They are not about Go Fund *Us*. Psychic numbing takes place when we look at what happens to many, in contrast to what happens to one. Recall the 1991 video of the Los Angelis police stomping Rodney King, or the photo of the Syrian child lying face down washed up on a Turkey beach. We need experience to believe something is true.

How can we draw attention to vague statements such as "inequality kills" or "early life lasts a lifetime," rather than the individual situations that our media focus on relentlessly? How do we overcome indifference or respond to apathy, namely the plight of a whole country such as the United States, which suffers from a huge health inequity? Mis-information plays a role, as we have seen with COVID-19 deniers. In George Orwell's *1984* the response was thought control.

Complacency is a sibling to indifference: A feeling of self-satisfaction especially when unaware of upcoming trouble. Health in the United States is getting worse. This shouldn't be happening.

Donating to philanthropic causes begs the question of charity's effectiveness. A better way is to emphasize science education and foster critical thinking in non-hierarchical and non-competitive environments. Craft effective stories. You will be praised for your prosocial ideas when your motives prevent you from benefitting financially or by gaining status from doing so. People look askance at self-promoters. Point out that humans are an altruistic species when it comes to group behavior. We are not a selfish species. A better world is possible.

Conclusion

Twenty years from now you will be more disappointed by the things that you didn't do than by what you did. What matters is not to know the world, but to change it. Start doing new things, and share your good ideas with me. Don't be missing in action. We must organize or die. I close with a poem from a 1980 book by Marge Piercy, *The Moon is Always Female:*

THE LOW ROAD

By Marge Piercy
What can they do
to you? Whatever they want.
They can set you up, they can

bust you, they can break
your fingers, they can
burn your brain with electricity,
blur you with drugs till you
can't walk, can't remember, they can
take your child, wall up
your lover. They can do anything
you can't stop them
from doing. How can you stop
them? Alone, you can fight,
you can refuse, you can
take what revenge you can
but they roll over you.

Two people can keep each other
sane, can give support, conviction,
love, massage, hope, sex.
Three people are a delegation,
a committee, a wedge. With four
you can play bridge and start
an organization. With six
you can rent a whole house,
eat pie for dinner with no
seconds and hold a fundraising party.
A dozen make a demonstration.
A hundred fill a hall.

A thousand have solidarity and your own newsletter;
ten thousand, power and your own paper;
A hundred thousand, your own media;
ten million, your own country.

It goes on one at a time.
it starts when you care
to act, it starts when you do
it again after they said *No*,
it starts when you say *We*
and know who you mean, and each
day you mean one more.

Questions to Consider and Discuss

1. What kinds of strategies for personal, group, national, and international action have not been presented here that should have been?
2. What world view or paradigm shapes your vision and action? Do you want to shift it slightly? How?

References

1. Wohlmuth E. The Overnight Guide to Public Speaking. New York, NY: Penguin Group; 1993.
2. Waitzkin H, Pérez A, Anderson M. Social Medicine and the Coming Transformation. New York, NY: Routledge; 2021.
3. Selwyn D, ed. At the Center of All Possibilities: Transforming Education for Our Children's Future. New York, NY: Peter Lang; 2022.
4. Bezruchka, S. Teaching Knowledge and Action to Promote Health Improvement: At the Center of All Possibilities: Transforming Education for Our Children's Future In Selwyn D, editor. New York, NY: Peter Lang; 2022.
5. Margolin J. Youth to Power: Your Voice and How to Use It. New York, NY: Hachette; 2020.
6. Alinsky SD. Rules for Radicals: A Practical Primer for Realistic Radicals. New York, NY: Vintage Books; 1989.
7. Chomsky N, Derber C. Chomsky for Activists. New York, NY: Routledge; 2021.
8. Martinson M, Su C, Minkler M. Contrasting Organizing Approaches: The "Alinsky Tradition" and Freirian Organizing Approaches In: Minkler M, Wakimoto P, editors. Community Organizing and Community Building for Health and Welfare. 4th ed. New Brunswick, NJ: Rutgers University Press; 2021. p. 76–85.
9. Freire P. Pedagogy of the Oppressed. New York, NY: Continuum; 2000.
10. Klein N. This Changes Everything: Capitalism vs. the Climate. New York, NY: Simon & Schuster; 2014.
11. Salerno BA. Sister Societies: Women's Antislavery Organizations in Antebellum America. DeKalb: Northern Illinois University Press; 2005.

Afterword

It's 2022 as I write these final words, and one question that is on everybody's mind is, are we near the beginning of the end of the COVID-19 viral blizzard? If, in 2019, someone had predicted that in a year or more the world would be devastated with a disease that did not exist at that time, you would almost certainly have discounted such nonsense. While experts had been predicting emerging infections for a long time, we have been lulled into a false sense of security from contagions.

The 1918 influenza pandemic killed many millions worldwide, mostly those of younger ages. Subsequent flu outbreaks in the 1950s and 60s killed older folk, but overall many fewer died during these epidemics than in the earlier one. Advances in medical care made populations more confident that whatever happened, we could cope, thanks to modern treatments.

The last half century has seen exponential technological change. Scientific, engineering, and technical advances have produced previously unimagined, incredibly powerful technology. As noted in Chapter 7, mobile phones put more computing power in our palms than got us to the moon in 1969. As a species, we seemed to be invincible. Given all the information, data, and health technology available to us, how did we get to today's situation?

At the end of 2019, a few news clips of a cluster of cases of pneumonia appeared in Wuhan, China. The World Health Organization (WHO) took notice in January 2020, around the same time that China shared the genetic sequence of a novel virus, SARS-CoV-2. By the end of January 2020, WHO declared the infection a Public Health Emergency of International Concern.

By then, the first reported U.S. cases had already appeared in nursing homes in Washington State. WHO declared COVID-19 a pandemic in March 2020, and U.S. government officials warned we could suffer over a hundred thousand possible deaths here. Yet the American President denied the crisis and cut financial backing for WHO, while scoffing at those who wore masks and railing against any efforts to close public spaces. Soon afterwards, however, U.S. government funding was made available for the rapid development of a vaccine for the coronavirus.

Deaths in the United States and rich countries mounted, and even more dire predictions circulated. Countries had very different responses to the pandemic.

East Asian countries did massive testing, contact tracing, and quarantining, thereby limiting its initial spread. The U.S. reaction lagged severely, and soon our COVID-19 death toll led the world.

By the end of 2020, just as the pandemic was at its height and the country sharply divided politically as a newly elected president prepared to assume power, two American pharmaceutical companies produced vaccines. Big Pharma typically does not invest in prevention (such as producing vaccines) or even cures, in comparison to investing in expensive drugs that maintain people with chronic conditions. But COVID-19 could be a windfall for Big Pharma. One of the two, Pfizer, estimated their profit margin from their vaccine could be on the order of 80%. Pfizer's strategy was to be the first to the market. As an incentive, the U.S. government paid Pfizer $2 billion for that initial batch. Pfizer cut similar deals with other rich countries. In early 2021, a massive vaccination campaign was launched. With people desperate, other governments paid Pfizer dearly for the product and for the extremely costly cold storage chain required to keep the vaccine effective. The vaccine appears to be the biggest revenue generating drug ever—yet those profits will not be returned to the public that funded its research, because Big Pharma retains the intellectual property rights—hence profits— of the drugs they develop with our tax dollars (1). Nevertheless, the government cost seemed worth it, as the effectiveness of the vaccine suggested we were at the beginning of the end.

How did we get to the COVIDian crisis? Recall the efforts described in Chapter 3 to go upstream to the source of a problem. Why do novel infections occur? SARS-CoV-2 may have come to us from bats in China. Why? For several reasons including, most importantly, we have destroyed natural wildlife habitats by massive deforestation, planting mono crops, and living closer and closer to wild environments. These practices vastly disrupted predator and prey relations. As human numbers on the earth increased rapidly, and we crowded together in cities, we ended up being easy prey for some creatures, including viruses. The virus also lives in other animal populations making eradication virtually impossible.

The acceptance of such knowledge is facing a crisis today, however, because our ability to concentrate and think critically is being eroded by the incredibly successful business of surveillance capitalism. Social media distracts us constantly and doesn't allow us to evaluate competing pieces of evidence. The end result is not just a rejection of critical thinking, but of scientific knowledge itself—such as the massive dismissal by a third of Americans of the very vaccine that supposedly could save their lives. Let's trace how we come to understand concepts.

Acceptance of scientific advances is slow, for the most part. At one point in history, we all knew the sun went around the earth. Then Copernicus postulated that the sun, rather than the earth, was at the center of the solar system. It took a few centuries before this idea was fully accepted. Occasionally a scientific theory, such as the power of the atom, led to the rapid development of something catastrophically important—the atomic bomb. That Manhattan Project took five years. Similarly, in 1957, when Russia launched a satellite, a space race ensued, leading to the moon landing in 1969. Details of some developments, like the bomb, are mostly kept secret from the public until they are visible and others garner public attention. The secrecy of some scientific research and advancements, and the lack of understanding of the scientific method, can lead some people to reject all science and the institutions that produce it.

Scientists and engineers usually begin their research by submitting proposals to public, private, and philanthropic institutions to obtain funding for their efforts. Such work takes years, and once the funds have been obtained and the research conducted, the results are submitted for publication in an academic journal. A lengthy peer-review process follows that may lead to publication (which may legitimize the findings) or the effort may be rejected (which means the findings are not circulated among the usual communication channels in the scientific community). As a result of this process, academia is full of strategies to get published so careers advance. Publish or perish is not just a quip to academics—it is the first rule of their positions.

Such a vetting process has not taken place with SARS-CoV-2 and COVID-19, however. The urgency of this new infection has led to many hypotheses and research studies presented on the internet without peer review. This production of public knowledge is not all science: "reality" can also be purchased on social media, so almost anyone can say just about anything about the pandemic and be heard. The public, already in a state of heightened fear and social distress, hears these constant, and often conflicting, reports and all too often believes that which conforms to their level of comfort—not the objective legitimacy of the findings.

To address this confusion and chaos, the U.S. Center for Disease Control and Prevention (CDC) and public health departments have produced a variety of conflicting guidelines and recommendations for dealing with the pandemic. Many of these called for limited physical contact and have affected the economy. The pressure to get commerce moving, despite many problems, has led to relaxation of efforts to limit spread of SARS-CoV-2. People are also tired of being on alert for so long. Pandemic fatigue has set in. One lesson from the current experience; pandemics end psychologically before they do biologically.

Our public health agencies had been massively defunded in the last decade or more. Lack of coordination among states in the United States and among countries further hampered efforts to contain the pandemic. In the United States, there is no formal decision-making process to guide policy. Public health experts are not those in charge. Consequently, many conflicting statements appear. Unofficially, the U.S. COVID-19 policy continues to be "no policy." However, vaccination continues to be seen as the savior.

The phrase "public health" in the United States in response to COVID has become associated with what some claim aim to limit personal freedoms, such as mandating masking and vaccinations. Whatever good image our public health system had in the public's eye has been severely tarnished in the eyes of many. Rebuilding public health's image here will be challenging.

Various forms of political systems, centered around capitalist economies, have been unable to deal with the pandemic. Market mechanisms failed us with the banking crisis in 2008–9, and required public bailouts for the rich bankers. Massive financial support has been necessary with the COVID-19 crisis. The levels of this support and mechanisms to mitigate the economic impact on households during this crisis have varied tremendously around the world, with the United States significantly behind what has been provided in many other rich nations. The so-called free market has failed us.

Tracking the number of cases and deaths has been difficult. Some agencies have suggested the reported deaths may be vast underestimates. The United States appears to lead in numbers of deaths (more than a million) with the global count, July 2022, at almost 6,500,000. China, where all this started, reported over 22,000 deaths to WHO, despite having a population five times that of the United States. Tracking overall deaths includes those from COVID as well as others. This allows recognizing excess deaths in the tallies, no matter what the cause.

Countries that had fared the best in keeping deaths from SARS-CoV-2 low initially appeared to be those where there is more trust in society, and in their governments. American faith in government is at an all-time low.

Several vaccines were initially developed to deal with the Wuhan strain that appeared to decrease deaths among elderly vaccinees. This strategy, vaccinating during the pandemic, may however, in part, be responsible for the development of novel SARS-CoV-2 variants, with the Omicron variants of 2022 being easily spread and causing significant concern throughout the world. Perhaps a variant will appear as contagious as Omicron and as serious as Delta. We are caught in a sprint between vaccines and variants—and who do you think is winning? This is a place we've never been before: the age of variants. Countries that had previously done well have seen COVID-19 surges with Omicron. The future is uncertain.

What might the best strategy be? To begin, practice humility. Recognize how little certainty there is regarding the COVID-19 pandemic. Lockdown policies leave essential workers exposed. I had the privilege of laptop work from home to limit my exposure. Poorer people did not have that option but had to expose themselves to infection. As expected, they have been hardest hit by the virus and suffered the most deaths. Older people, especially those housed in care facilities and suffering from chronic illnesses, were quite vulnerable. Targeted surveillance and limiting close contact in those situations made sense.

Might we have embarked on the wrong *global* strategy to control SARS-CoV-2? A Belgian vaccinologist, Dr. Geert Vanden Bossche, pointed out in March 2021 that trying to immunize during a raging pandemic would lead to the proliferation of viral variants. Dr. Vanden Bossche wrote a letter to WHO explaining how the immunization program could derail efforts to control the pandemic globally. His second call to WHO in December 2021 presented more scientific evidence of this possibly faulty strategy. Some who were initially very skeptical are now coming around to considering his point of view. One recent piece of evidence is the apparent low rates of cases in Africa, where there has been little vaccination and where many people have relatively high levels of antibodies to SARS-CoV-2. In other words, they have become infected but not sick, perhaps because of innate immunity after exposure to that or related viruses. There is no consensus among experts here. More infectious variants may evolve that may not necessarily be more virulent as the virus wants to propagate and won't be successful if too many infected die. Vanden Bossche's ideas should be considered(2).

Today we live in a surrealistic world. People who have already had COVID-19 get re-infected as do those who have had the vaccine and been boosted. This pandemic is not behaving as would be expected from studies of other viral contagions. One Nobel Prize winning virologist (Luc Montagnier), warned that the COVID-19 vaccine could cause variants. Why is there such controversy? Is it different from that regarding the sun rather than the earth as the center of the solar system? Recall that a quarter of U.S. adults believe the sun orbits the earth.

Scientists studying the effects of SARS-CoV-2 are specialists who work in very circumscribed research areas. There is less support for a multi-disciplinary perspective where concepts from various scientific areas are synthesized to give a big-picture or upstream point of view. The arguments in this book linking economic inequality and compromised early life represent this generalist, rather than specialized, point of view. Vanden Bossche presents such a perspective as he integrates concepts of evolutionary biology, virology, vaccinology, and clinical medicine (albeit he is a veterinarian). Although he may be right, his views are discounted.

Health consequences for the United States may be those of a triple recession (3). One is an economic recession, which began before the pandemic. Reports of a recovery abound but surges in inflation call that into question. Secondly, we are facing a social or social capital recession. There is more loneliness and isolation than before with attendant increases in anxiety and depression. Long term we can expect to see suicides and deaths of despair climb. With rising mortality, we are living shorter, less-happy lives. The third recession is in education and human capital. School closures and remote learning have contributed to loss of educational opportunities. Poorer folk, those lower down the socioeconomic ladder, have borne the brunt of this type of recession. This will likely lead to reduced child and adolescent cognitive development. For 2020–21 life expectancy drops in the United States have exceeded those in other rich nations(4). Long term, we can expect life expectancy and other mortality measures in the United States to remain worse than those in many other nations.

There are more articles in the media about how many people die in this country that wouldn't if we had the health of other rich nations. One report on this injustice synthesizes much information and has links to many useful sources(5).

Past responses to economic recessions or depressions have included social spending, the creation of a safety net, and other national policies. Economic inequality is linked to recessions in social and human capital. Besides reducing economic inequality as this book has proposed, a targeted response to those most affected, those poorer, makes sense in the short term.

We lack critical scientific thinking, both among experts and among the general population. A distrust of scientific knowledge does not bode well for creating the global action plan that is required to deal with the pandemic. Effective ways of dealing with a science denier require establishing trust with her or him, showing respect and discussing rather than attacking (6).

Hospitals and medical care have been seriously disrupted in many places around the world. We have seen that medical care treats cells and organs but not populations. Nevertheless, sick people need care. Burnout among those providing medical services is raging. Staffing issues abound. One of the most critical medical resources in short supply today is hope. Can we develop effective drug treatments or cures for COVID-19? Yes, if we recognize that hope is a discipline. We must maintain optimism of the will. Small steps, taken together, will lead to big strides.

Meanwhile, promising new political strategies are becoming effective. Worker strikes are happening. Unionization is growing. Many are quitting meaningless jobs. Solidarity economies are flourishing, as people work together for common needs. We are recognizing that capitalism is mostly useful for protecting those who have too much and not the rest of us.

Thomas Piketty in his *Brief History of Equality* argues for having a system of participatory socialism and paying reparations for the ravages of the colonial and neo-colonial past (7). William Darity presents one strategy for U.S. reparations that would take excess White wealth in the United States today and transfer it so African Americans who had one slave ancestor would receive enough to eradicate the racial wealth gap(8).

We argue that the root cause of our current troubles is the vastly increasing economic inequality. As the pandemic plunged many into poverty, pandemic profiteering raised the wealth of a tiny few to obscene levels, with the ten richest men *doubling* their wealth from March 2020 to November 2021. These ten men now own more than the bottom 3.1 billion people on earth. If their combined wealth was piled up in freshly minted U.S. dollar bills, they would reach halfway to the moon. Many studies link income inequality to COVID-19 deaths, yet our response to COVID-19 has only escalated this inequality. We have learned that inequality kills. If we don't deal with this fundamental problem, we can be sure of more misfortune.

Much will be written, filmed, and discussed about the COVID-19 pandemic. This event must lead to serious questioning of how humans inhabit the planet, how we treat each other, and what needs to be done to improve not only the health and well-being of our species but also that of other creatures large and small, and the earth on which we live. The entomologist E.O. Wilson noted that "We are drowning in information, while starving for wisdom. The world henceforth will be run by synthesizers, people able to put together the right information at the right time, think critically about it, and make important choices wisely(9)."

We may not be at the beginning of the end of the pandemic, but we are at the end of the beginning. Will this virus become endemic like influenza? There is too much mud on the crystal ball to tell. How about the climate crisis, the major emergency affecting our human survival?

Are we entering the pandemicene as a sequel to the anthropocene, the era where humans exercised immense destructive power over the earth(10)? Nearly all pandemics start with an infectious agent making a jump from another animal species to us. The pandemicene may be the planet's response to the massive global warming our species has caused. COVID-19 is the tip of the iceberg. As the iceberg melts the heat wave may release a fiery future of untold infectious agents, mostly viruses, that interact with our native, naive immune system(11). This immunity has likely been detrimentally affected by our less than effective SARS-CoV-2 vaccines.

The world is in a precarious state for humanity at present. The political right has more clout than the fragmented political left. Our current global delivery chain is very unstable with food supply chains severely disrupted. We are in the midst of an upheaval in how the future will be structured. Each political and economic system in human history has had a beginning and an end. A few hundred years ago, feudalism's demise gave birth to capitalism. Capitalism in its current form will also end at some point. What will replace it is unclear, but it will hopefully have socialist elements that protect workers and ordinary people from the current wounds of austerity. And we will need to create a new world order to sustain life on the planet.

By considering economic inequality, together with the lack of support for early life, as the root causes of poor health among nations, we can take action. The steps outlined in Chapter 10 are the "medicine" we need. These steps have proven to be effective elsewhere. Apply as directed and as often as you can.

References

1. Nichols J. Coronavirus Criminals and Pandemic Profiteers: Accountability for Those Who Caused the Crisis. London: Verso; 2022.
2. Vanden Bossche G. Poor Virus-Neutralizing Capacity in Highly C-19 Vaccinated Populations Could Soon Lead to a Fulminant Spread of Sars-CoV-2 Super Variants That Are Highly Infectious and Highly Virulent in Vaccinees While Being Fully Resistant to All Existing and Future Spike-Based C-19 Vaccines. Belgium: Voice for Science and Solidarity; 2022 March 30.
3. Kim D. Minimizing Public Health Consequences of the COVID-19 Pandemic: Let's Consider the Threat of a Triple Recession. The Lancet Regional Health – Americas. 2022;8: 100176.
4. Van Noorden, R. COVID death tolls: scientists acknowledge errors in WHO estimates. Nature. June 2021. Available from: https://www.nature.com/articles/d41586-022-01526-0 [accessed July 22, 2022].
5. Yong, E. America Was in an Early-Death Crisis Long Before COVID. July 21, 2022. The Atlantic Monthly. Available from: https://www.theatlantic.com/health/archive/2022/07/us-life-span-mortality-rates/670591/

6. McIntyre LC. How to Talk to a Science Denier: Conversations With Flat Earthers, Climate Deniers, and Others Who Defy Reason. Cambridge, Massachusetts: The MIT Press; 2021.

7. Piketty, T, Rendall S. A Brief History of Equality. Cambridge, MA: The Belknap Press of Harvard University Press; 2022.

8. Darity Jr, WA, Mullen, AK. From Here to Equality: Reparations for Black Americans in the Twenty-First Century. Chapel Hill, NC: UNC Press Books; 2020.

9. Wilson EO. Consilience: The Unity of Knowledge. New York, NY: Knopf; 1998.

10. Yong E. We Created the 'Pandemicene'. The Atlantic Monthly. 2022 April 28.

11. Carlson CJ, Albery GF, Merow C, Trisos CH, Zipfel CM, Eskew EA, et al. Climate change increases cross-species viral transmission risk. Nature. 2022;607(7919):555–62.

Index